Advanced Praise for
Breast Cancer Facts, Myths, and Controversies

"Dr. Finkel's book comes at such an important time when there is a lot of information and misinformation related to breast cancer. This scientifically based book helps to clarify the complexities of breast cancer screening for the layperson. It also provides helpful information for patients about treatment options, support groups, and strategies to cope and thrive with breast cancer."

—Dr. Rulla Tamimi, Professor of Population Health Sciences,
Weill Cornell Medicine

"Ambitious and engaging, Professor Finkel provides an exceptional overview of the complexities of breast cancer. Finkel's personal experience is elegantly woven throughout and provides critical insight, from screening to treatment. An essential text for anyone looking to better understand the field."

—Eloise May O'Donnell, Senior Research Manager,
Weill Cornell Medicine

Breast Cancer Facts, Myths, and Controversies

Understanding Current Screenings and Treatments

Madelon L. Finkel, PhD

Public Health Issues and Developments

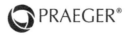 PRAEGER®

An Imprint of ABC-CLIO, LLC
Santa Barbara, California • Denver, Colorado

Library of Congress Cataloging-in-Publication Data

Names: Finkel, Madelon Lubin, 1949- author.
Title: Breast cancer facts, myths, and controversies : understanding
  current screenings and treatments / Madelon L. Finkel.
Description: Santa Barbara, California : ABC-CLIO, [2021] | Series: Public
  health issues and developments | Includes bibliographical references and
  index.
Identifiers: LCCN 2020048191 (print) | LCCN 2020048192 (ebook) | ISBN
  9781440875137 (hardcover) | ISBN 9781440875144 (ebook)
Subjects: LCSH: Breast—Cancer—Treatment. | Breast—Cancer—Risk factors.
Classification: LCC RC280.B8 F557 2021 (print) | LCC RC280.B8 (ebook) |
  DDC 616.99/449—dc23
LC record available at https://lccn.loc.gov/2020048191
LC ebook record available at https://lccn.loc.gov/2020048192

ISBN: 978-1-4408-7513-7 (print)
      978-1-4408-7514-4 (ebook)

25 24 23 22 21   1 2 3 4 5

This book is also available as an eBook.

Praeger
An Imprint of ABC-CLIO, LLC

ABC-CLIO, LLC
147 Castilian Drive
Santa Barbara, California 93117
www.abc-clio.com

This book is printed on acid-free paper ∞

Manufactured in the United States of America

This book is dedicated to my beloved mother, Lorraine Lubin, and to all other women diagnosed with breast cancer. My mother's strength in coping with her disease never wavered, and she lived her life to its fullest, even during chemo treatments. She truly was a profile in courage for her daughters and granddaughters.

Contents

Preface

There has been so much written about breast cancer over the past decades, making it sometimes difficult for one to stay abreast of all the new surgical, radiological, and medical advances that have been made. While breast cancer continues to be the most commonly diagnosed cancer among women around the world, the good news is that breast cancer deaths have decreased substantially over time. This decline is attributed to improvements in treatment and early detection. The American Cancer Society estimates that there are more than 3.6 million breast cancer survivors in the United States, and hopefully the number will continue to increase.

Whether one develops breast cancer or not depends on many factors. Some women are at higher risk than others, and survival also differs, depending on an individual's genetic, demographic, and clinical factors. That being said, having one or more risk factors does not automatically imply that an individual will develop breast cancer. All it means is that the risk of breast cancer is higher among those with risk factors compared to those who have no risk factors. But, in fact, 85% of breast cancers occur in women who have no risk factors. It is complicated!

This book presents a comprehensive overview of breast cancer facts, myths, and controversies. I made sure to include the most up-to-date, scientifically rigorous published studies on the topics, and I discuss the findings and implications of the large-scale clinical trials on mammogram screening that were conducted decades ago. No large-scale clinical trials have been conducted in recent times.

I was motivated to write the book for many reasons, including experiencing firsthand my mother's bout with breast cancer, her years in remission, and the cancer's return 10 years after the initial diagnosis. I found my training in epidemiology to be helpful in understanding the course of the disease, but woefully lacking in helping me to cope with the emotional roller coaster of her cancer treatments. Many of my friends who are breast cancer survivors would ask about treatment options, and I realized that navigating the system and understanding the pros and cons of these options was daunting. This book is an effort to explain the potential benefits and harms of existing and new therapeutics as well as the controversy surrounding the potential benefits and harms of mammography screening.

While new therapeutics hold great promise, they may not be uniformly effective for every woman. What may be the most appropriate drug for one person may not be for another. Precision medicine offers great hope to tailor treatment to an individual, but determining who will benefit from specific treatments is complex and somewhat imprecise. As we learn more about the short-term and long-term effects of each type of treatment, we inch closer to increasing survival from breast cancer. My hope is that the book will serve as a guide in understanding the complexities of breast cancer and the treatments for this disease.

Breast cancer screening has been touted as the "best" means to identify a tumor in its early stages and improve survival. Does mammography deliver on its promise? In our efforts to screen for early disease, are we doing more harm than good? To what extent does mammography detect something that would not have caused a problem if left alone? The book provides up-to-date information to address these and other questions.

There are literally tens of thousands of articles that have been published on the topic. I have tried to present the "best evidence" in a clear, concise manner so that the layperson can understand the issues and controversies. A helpful glossary of terms is included at the end of the book, as are breast cancer screening guidelines posted by leading organizations.

Chapter 1 presents an historical overview of how art, literature, and society viewed the female breast. Over the course of history, psychiatrists, politicians, pornographers, religious leaders, artists, and writers have either rhapsodized or vilified the female breast. Marilyn Yalom, author of *The History of the Breast*, writes that the female breast is, at varying times, sources of wonder, pleasure, sensual delight, pain, humiliation, and anguish. The chapter concludes with a discussion of the different types of breast disease (benign and malignant) to illustrate how complex breast diseases are.

Worldwide breast cancer is one of the most common cancers in women. That being said, not every woman will develop breast cancer over the course of her lifetime. Who is most at risk for breast cancer? What factors contribute to an increased risk of developing breast cancer? Chapter 2 presents a detailed overview of factors that have been shown to raise the risk of developing breast cancer. However, it is important to note that not every person with one or several risk factors will develop breast cancer. Indeed, many women with no risk factors are diagnosed with the disease. There are many factors that may contribute to the development of breast cancer, and the likelihood or odds of getting the disease is complex.

Screening for disease is not a new concept and is today one of the most basic tools of public health and preventive medicine. Chapter 3 presents the principles and purpose of screening. Screening is done not only to detect a disease or condition but also to improve survival. Screening is designed to identify disease at an early stage (early detection), which should contribute to the individual to live longer because of early detection and treatment. Potential harms of screening are presented, including false-positive and false-negative results. Screening may also lead to overdiagnosis and overtreatment.

The pros and cons of screening for different types of cancer are presented in chapter 4. While not every type of cancer would be appropriate for screening (i.e., ovarian cancer), screening for lung, breast, colorectal, prostate, and cervical cancer is recommended. Chapter 5 presents an overview of advances in breast cancer detection, especially the development of mammography. Over the past two decades, there have been exciting advances in breast cancer detection technology, including new ways to image the breast and new detection strategies aimed at finding distinctive "molecular signatures" of a premalignant or malignant breast tumor. Highly sophisticated technologies permit a more precise way to detect tumors and lesions at an early stage. These technologies are discussed in detail.

Breast cancer and mammography are synonymous in the public's mind. Although it has its limitations, mammography remains the most cost-effective, safe, and economic means of population-based screening for breast cancer. Yet, it is not without controversy. Chapters 6 reviews breast cancer screening guidelines for specific population groups: younger women <40 years; older women >70 years; women of different racial/ethnic groups; lesbian, gay, and bisexual women; and women with disabilities. A complicating factor is that there are different, even conflicting, guidelines regarding mammography screening. Although all support mammography screening, the guidelines vary in the recommended age at which to begin screening. Should one start screening at age 40? 45? 50? The answer depends on so many different factors. In point of fact, it is up to the individual woman in consultation with her doctor to make a decision about when and how frequently to have a mammogram.

Further complicating the issue, the long-term effectiveness of mammogram screening and its effect on survival, in particular, are subject to differences of opinion despite the fact that these opinions and recommendations are based on the same data sets! Everyone is looking at the same large-scale studies but arriving at slightly different interpretations of the study results. Chapter 7 presents an overview of the major breast cancer screening clinical trials. The mammogram debate is far from settled, which leaves the individual woman in a position where she will have to make a decision based on her perceived risks of breast cancer. The epidemiological studies and clinical trials are impersonal in that they rely on data from thousands of women. An individual woman's decision is much more emotional and personal.

Chapter 8 presents a comprehensive overview of advances in treatment (medical, surgical, and radiological) for breast cancer. Advances in adjuvant systemic therapy (chemotherapy), endocrine (hormonal) therapy, and biological immunotherapy/targeted therapy are discussed, including an explanation of estrogen and progesterone receptors, selective estrogen receptor modulators (SERMs), and HER2-positive breast cancer. Pharmaceutical therapies are used to treat different types of breast cancer (i.e., tamoxifen, herceptin, and aromatase inhibitors). Treatment options are proliferating not just for early-stage breast cancer but also for advanced metastatic cancer. The chapter makes it clear that there is no treatment option that is the "right" or "only" one. Treatment will vary depending on a number of factors, including the histological type of the cancer; the stage, and tumor size and location; how fast the cancer cells are growing; lymph node involvement; if the tumor is dependent on hormones and if so which ones; risk of recurrence; individual's age; and menopausal status.

Cancer is a heterogeneous catchall term to denote a malignant growth resulting from the division of abnormal cells in an uncontrolled way in the body. As chapter 8 makes clear, one size does not fit all. Cancer biology has advanced so rapidly, making precision or targeted medicine a reality. Targeted therapy is a much more precise approach to treatment, taking into account the unique situation in one patient, rather than generalizing treatments to fit all patients. Chapter 9 presents a description of targeted cancer therapy and the hope and promises it holds for cancer patients.

In addition to the exciting developments in cancer biology, there are other types of treatment that are used frequently by many patients: complementary, alternative, and integrated medicine (CAM). CAM options and therapies should not be viewed as a substitute or replacement for conventional treatments; rather they can be used along with conventional treatments. Chapter 10 presents an overview of the types and effectiveness of common CAM therapies.

A diagnosis of any cancer signifies an uncertain future filled with medical procedures, tests, and treatments, each with its own set of side effects and unknowns. Many breast cancer patients going through treatment describe themselves as being on a roller coaster. Changes in behavior and mood are common. Many women experience a host of psychological symptoms at some point during the course of treatment and posttreatment, including but not limited to sleep disturbance, fatigue, stress, anxiety, irritability, inability to cope, sadness, and depression. Feelings of loss of control can be upending and upsetting. Coping with breast cancer is an important, integral part of cancer treatment, and Chapter 11 talks about the importance of support networks, coping strategies, and why psycho-oncology is viewed as an integral component of cancer treatment.

Breast cancer patients have a diverse range of preferences regarding how active a role they wish to play when discussing and choosing treatment options. A good doctor-patient relationship is built on an open, honest foundation to permit shared decision-making. Chapter 12 explores the issues in shared decision-making and doctor-patient communication. Shared decision-making requires good listening skills for both parties. Each patient should be treated as an individual, as some individuals will want to know as much as possible while others may not. Some may want to be an active participant in decision-making while others may not. Physicians need to appreciate the range of patient and family needs in order to create a healthy doctor-patient relationship and must take care not to misjudge patient preferences.

The final chapter stresses the importance of support groups for patients undergoing cancer treatment as well as for those in remission. The message is that "You Are Not Alone." Chapter 13 is provided as a reference guide of organizations offering a wide variety of support groups for cancer patients. There are so many opportunities to reach out for help, advice, and support. All one has to do is ask!

Those who read this book should sense a note of optimism. Substantial advances in breast cancer research and medical technology enable those diagnosed with breast cancer today to live for many years, if not decades, after receiving the diagnosis. Many women will go into remission. Screening, despite its controversies, is still one of the best ways to detect early-stage tumors. More women are breast cancer survivors today than ever before. My mother lived over 15 active years after her mastectomy and chemotherapy. In fact, in her early sixties, she climbed not only the Himalayas but also the Peruvian Andes. In her late sixties, when her cancer recurred, she underwent another round of chemotherapy. Refusing to let her disease get the best of her, she managed to hike in the ruins of Petra (Jordan) with her daughter and granddaughter—in between chemo treatments! This book is dedicated to her and to all the women diagnosed with breast cancer.

Acknowledgments

Many thanks to my colleague Eloise O'Donnell, MPH, who spent countless hours reading each chapter and providing excellent suggestions as to how to improve the text. Her support and encouragement is much appreciated. Sincere thanks to my friend Marsha Gordon, a breast cancer survivor, who shared her most personal thoughts and feelings with me about her being told that she has breast cancer and her coping with chemo and radiation treatments. She is happily in remission over a decade later. To my daughter, Rebecca Finkel, who proofread the chapters and provided insightful comments, I say "Thank you." You are my biggest supporter and motivator!

CHAPTER ONE

The Female Breast: Its Image and Function through the Ages

Over the course of history, psychiatrists, psychologists, religious leaders, politicians, pornographers, artists, and writers have either rhapsodized or vilified the female breast. Marilyn Yalom, author of *The History of the Breast*, writes that the female breast is, at varying times, a source of wonder, pleasure, sensual delight, pain, humiliation, and anguish.[1] The female body, clothed and unclothed, and especially the female breast, the primary biological function of which is to produce milk to feed a baby, has been for many centuries not only a symbol of femininity, fertility, motherhood, and beauty but also one of eroticism and sexuality. Many women regard their breasts not only as a sign of femininity but also as an important component to their sexual attractiveness.

It is through literature and art that we gain a descriptive and visual understanding of how societies through the ages have portrayed and perceived the female breast. Greek mythology speaks of the Amazons, the fierce all-woman warrior society governed by a queen. The Amazons, it is said, cut off their right breast in order to be better able to draw back a bow to shoot an arrow. The Kama Sutra of Vatsyayana, the ancient Indian Sanskrit text on sexuality, eroticism, and emotional fulfillment in life, is considered to be the first written work on human sexuality. In this ancient Indian Sanskrit text, the female breast figures prominently in descriptions of love making.

The female breast also served to symbolize freedom and resistance. Marianne, for example, has been the national symbol of the French Republic since the time of the French revolution. She is regarded as a symbol against the old ruling monarchy and is meant to represent the personification of liberty, equality, fraternity, and reason. The French painter Eugène Delacroix's

19th-century masterpiece, *Liberty Leading the People*, which commemorates the July Revolution of 1830 that ended the reign of King Charles X of France, shows a barefoot and bare-breasted Liberty (i.e., Marianne) as both an allegorical goddess-figure and a robust woman of the people.

The Female Breast as Portrayed in Art

Portrayal of the female with partially covered or uncovered breasts is ubiquitous in all forms of art, including painting, sculpture, drawing, sketches, mosaics, photography, ceramics, and film. Throughout the ages, and in all cultures, depiction of the female breast also conveys a sense of the social norms and mores of the time and place. Rock carvings and sacred statues with breasts date from 15,000 BC, and the sculptures of female figures that date from the Stone Age (8700 to 2000 BCE) are endowed with highly exaggerated breasts and ample hips.

The female breast is depicted in Egyptian papyri dating from the 18th dynasty (1550 to 1292 BCE), but only for female deities who are breastfeeding pharaohs, perhaps serving as "proof" of the woman's divine status. The representation of the female breast in papyri, however, was essentially done to convey motherhood and fertility and not for any sexual or erotic reason. For example, the Egyptian goddess Isis, worshiped as the ideal, fertile mother, is often shown nursing her son Horus, the falcon-headed god who today is one of the most commonly used symbols of Egypt. Horus is considered to be one of the most significant of the ancient Egyptian deities, and the ancient Egyptians believed that the pharaoh was the "living Horus."

The ancient Greeks focused on the male body in their art and sculptures, with athletic nude men portrayed as the ultimate ideal of beauty. The few sculpted female nudes depict Aphrodite, the Greek goddess of sexual love and beauty, bare breasted with her hand modestly covering her genitals. Other female Greek deities depicted in ancient Greek art are dressed, with breasts concealed under the drapes of their robes. In contrast, ancient Roman frescoes, mosaics, and sculpture depict well-endowed females. During the Chola dynasty in south India (9th to 13th century), statues and paintings of the goddess Parvati, the Indian goddess of fertility, clearly show a female figure with extremely rounded breasts and pointy nipples.

There are very few images of the female breast in art in the Middle Ages (AD 476 to 1453), almost all being depictions of the Virgin Mary breastfeeding baby Jesus (e.g., *The Nursing Madonna, Virgo Lactans,* or *Madonna Lactans*), as a motif for life and religiousness. European Renaissance art, painting, sculpture, architecture, music, and literature produced during the 14th to 16th century marks the transition from the medieval period to the Early Modern Age. Whereas medieval art was mostly flat and dark depicting human religious figures, the Renaissance style (especially in the 15th and

16th centuries) emphasized nature, beauty, shadow, and light. Sandro Botticelli's *Birth of Venus* painting (mid-1480s) is considered to be the first non-religious nude painted since classical antiquity.

Great masters of the Renaissance, including Leonardo di ser Piero da Vinci, Michelangelo di Lodovico Buonarroti Simoni, and Raffaello Sanzio da Urbino (known as Raphael), often depicted bare-breasted women in their paintings. A prime example is the Sistine Chapel, built in 1473 to 1481 by the architect Giovanni dei Dolci for Pope Sixtus IV, famous for its Renaissance frescoes by Michelangelo. The ceiling is adorned with paintings of women with one or both breasts uncovered; however, this Christian religious work of art depicts the breast in a maternal form and not in a sexual or erotic way.

The Flemish painter Peter Paul Rubens (1577 to 1640), in particular, is well known for portraying women in a sensual yet natural way, depicting robust, buxom women with less than perfect bodies. Many years later, Francisco de Goya y Lucientes's *The Nude Maja* (1797) shocked society by his use of a model in a contemporary setting, showing pubic hair rather than the smooth perfection of goddesses and nymphs.

During the same time period but in different parts of the world, symbolic and erotic images of the female breast also were evident. During the Edo period in Japan (1630 to 1868), shunga art depicted very explicit and graphic sexual encounters and were widely popular at the time, despite the many censorship programs and punishments the government implemented.[2]

In 19th-century European art, exposed breasts were acceptable, while a woman's bared legs, ankles, or shoulders were considered risqué. Baring one's breast (i.e., going topless) was socially normal in many indigenous societies. That is, in many African tribes and South Pacific islands women going about their daily chores bare breasted was considered to be culturally acceptable. Artists captured the beauty of the female form in non-Western societies, most notably the late 19th-century painter Eugène Henri Paul Gauguin. His masterpiece, *Two Tahitian Women*, is illustrative of the depiction of native topless women.

The 20th-century depiction of the female nude perhaps reflects the changing norms of the time. For example, Henri Matisse's *Blue Nude* (1907) shocked the French public when it was exhibited, but this work had a strong effect on another contemporary artist, Pablo Picasso. Pablo Picasso's *Les Demoiselles d'Avignon* (1907) is a large oil painting that portrays five nude female prostitutes in a brothel. Years later, 20th-century artist Lucien Freud's powerful nude portraits focused on the male and female anatomy in great detail.

Of course, there are many more examples of the female form in paintings and sculpture as well as in other art forms such as photography, which has a rich history of capturing the female nude, but these will not be discussed here. Suffice it to say that through all forms of art, one can observe a snapshot of the cultural and sexual norms of the time and place.

The Female Breast in Fashion

Art, in many ways, is a reflection of society, and similarly fashion has been, and continues to be, an important part of society and culture. Throughout the ages, women's garments served to either accentuate or conceal their breasts. Women's garments and devices (e.g., the corset) covered, constrained, and revealed breasts. Ever-changing fashion styles gyrated from covering up the breast, to seductively exposing a significant portion of it, to "letting it all hang out." In 2500 BCE, warrior Minoan women on the Greek isle of Crete are depicted as wearing a bra-resembling garment/corset that shoved the bare breasts up and out of their clothing, which served to make the breast more visible despite being wrapped in some type of garment. This arrangement probably had an erotic connotation because of its effect to accentuate the breasts. Historical depictions of that time also show that ancient Greek women used a small band of material wrapped around the breasts (the *apodesme*—breast band) to prevent the breasts from moving; ancient Roman women, too, adopted the apodesme in their garments.

Whereas during the early Middle Ages in Europe (AD 500 to 1000) women wore a free-form, chemise-type garment that offered no support to the breasts, by the 13th and 14th centuries, women wore a straight, tubular bodice that served to completely flatten their breasts. This design was primarily for function rather than emphasis on form. In England during the reign of King Henry VI (1421 to 1471), "baring the breasts" was considered disrespectful. King Henry banned all depictions of breasts, and women had to conceal them with bands and clothes.[3] An early version of the corset, made of whalebone and steel rods (which sounds perfectly uncomfortable), was designed to ensure the constraint of the breasts. However, décolletage was very fashionable during the Renaissance.

In Victorian England (1837 to 1901), despite its strict codes of social conduct, women's clothing was paradoxically designed to emphasize both the breasts and hips. While women were expected to cover their bodies, the style of dress was deliberately provocatively designed to emphasize and expose as much of the breasts as possible. The corset was an essential element of female fashion during this era and was the dominant undergarment of support and restraint for the next 350 years!

It was not until the early 1900s that women's clothing became more free form in style. To accommodate the new look, the corset evolved into a more natural undergarment. Shoulder straps, rather than rigid staves, served to support the breasts and were referred to as a "brassiere." In 1889, Mme. Herminie Cadolle devised a garment called the Bien-Être (meaning "well-being"), which connected with sashes over the shoulders to the corset in the back.[4] "Brassiere," which comes from the old French word for upper arm, was first coined in 1907 by the *Vogue* magazine.[5] Prior to that, brassieres were known by the French term *soutien-gorge*, or "throat support" or "breast support."

During World War I, the U.S. War Industries Board requested that women stop buying corsets in order to conserve metal for military purposes. This action not only helped make available tons of metal for use toward the war effort but also liberated women from this tight-fitting garment. Fortuitously, prior to the start of the War, in 1913, socialite Mary Phelps Jacob and her maid, Marie, devised a backless bra made from two handkerchiefs, ribbon, and cord. This lightweight, soft brassiere, albeit without cups, was the first modern-day prototype bra, which was intended to flatten the breasts rather than enhance them, creating an androgynous look. This design was immediately popular with the women at the time. Several years later, Mrs. Jacob sold her business to Warner Brothers Corset Company for a princely sum of $1,500. The early prototype bra gave limited support, and the sizing was imprecise. In the 1930s, the Warners devised A to D cup measurements to remedy this situation. The Warners made over $15 million over the ensuing decades by selling this garment.[6]

During the 1930s and 1940s, the changing views of the female body led to a dramatic shift away from the flat-chested look to a more buxom look. The new, all-elastic bra enhanced the breast, showing off a woman's curves. Hollywood helped create the glamorous image of full-busted movie stars. The sweater-girl look portrayed by the actress Lana Turner and others, as well as the sensuous pin-up poster girl, for example, set the look and the style so popular at the time. To enable less-endowed women to create a more full-figured look, falsies and the pushup bra were marketed.

The Female Breast as a Sex Symbol

Large, voluptuous breasts became synonymous with sex appeal, and sexy imagery was still favored by Hollywood movie directors in the 1950s. Marilyn Monroe most notably represented the ideal of beauty and femininity that was prevalent in the 1950s and 1960s. However, the female liberation movement of the 1960s unleashed expressions of feminism of a different sort. For some, this included not wearing a bra. Ironically, as women were seeking different expressions of feminism and liberation, *Playboy* magazine and other similar male-oriented publications continued to showcase the female anatomy. Also, the Barbie™ doll, introduced at the 1959 American Toy Fair in New York City, was characterized by large and protruding breasts on a thin and curvaceous body, idealizing the way a woman should look. In its first year, 300,000 Barbie dolls were sold. Barbie probably influenced many young girls' thoughts about body image and fashion, but attaining such a look was probably only possible from plastic surgery.

From the 1970s on, the bra was redesigned to provide comfort as well as to accent the breasts. Falsies and pads could be inserted in the bra to create a more full-bodied look. It was the pop star Madonna, in the 1990s, who showed that the bra need not be hidden under clothes. She and other media stars created a new look for the bra, and many women, famous or not, followed by wearing a lacey and frilly bustier as a fashion statement. The media continued to highlight full-busted women in movies, TV, and videos. Full-sized breasts were still synonymous with sex appeal and beauty.

As fashion and the media continued to focus on the female breast, many women in the 1980s and 1990s elected to have plastic surgery to enhance their appearance. Breast implants and breast augmentation surgery were embraced not only by models and movie stars but also by "ordinary" women. For those less inclined to undergo surgery, the uplift Wonderbra helped create the look of full-figured bosom.

The breast as a sex symbol, a symbol of eroticism, prevailed during the latter part of the 20th century. At the same time, however, the increase in incidence of breast cancer heightened awareness that the breast is a part of the body that could become diseased. Breast cancer, benign and malignant breast disease, treatment options, breast self-examination, and mammography were topics that were openly discussed and debated. In 1974, First Lady Bette Ford went public about her breast cancer and radical mastectomy. Two weeks after Ms. Ford's surgery, Happy Rockefeller, wife of Vice President Nelson Rockefeller, underwent a double mastectomy. These high-profile women helped to bring breast cancer out of the shadows and publicly raise awareness of this disease.

In order to have a better understanding of breast disease and the risk factors for breast cancer, it is important to know about the anatomy of the breast.

The Anatomy of the Breast

Breast tissue is composed of several elements: lobules (glandular tissue that contains cells that make and secrete milk), ducts (passageways that carry milk from the lobules to the nipple), fat (fatty tissue that surrounds the ducts and lobules), connective tissue (rough, fibrous strands that surround and support the breast), lymphatic vessels (carry clear fluid that contains immune system cells), and lymph nodes (part of the lymphatic system, a component of the body's immune system) (see figure 1.1). Breast tissue, which remains dormant until puberty when hormonal changes result in breast development, consists of glandular tissues (lobules and ducts) and stromal or supporting tissues (fatty and fibrous connective tissues). Any of these tissues can undergo changes that can result in either benign or malignant breast disease.

During a woman's reproductive years, monthly menstrual cycles cause the breast to swell, in some cases causing discomfort and pain. During pregnancy and lactation, the breast ducts and lobules multiply, and during the premenstrual years, breast tissue is generally dense. In menopause, there is a drop in hormonal stimulation, causing the glandular tissues to shrink and the breast to become more fatty and less dense. For many women, these

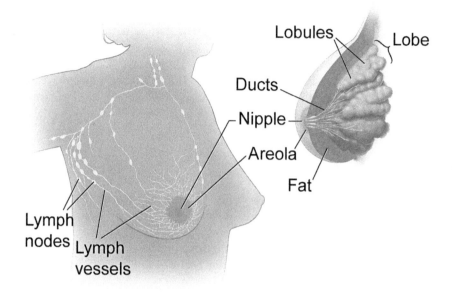

Figure 1.1 Breast anatomy. (Don Bliss [Illustrator], National Cancer Institute)

breast changes usually pose no problems. For others, however, symptoms such as swelling and/or tenderness, breast pain, or nipple discharge may occur. Although these symptoms do not automatically mean that something is wrong, a physician should be consulted and the condition evaluated.

Noncancerous Breast Disease

Benign breast conditions (noncancerous breast disease) do not generally increase the risk of breast cancer. While some conditions may not cause any symptoms and may be found only during a routine physical exam or routine screening mammography, others may be painful and have palpable lumps or masses. Generalized breast lumpiness, sometimes described as nodular, can often be felt in the area around the nipple and areola as well as in the upper-outer part of the breast. These lumps are common but are not life threatening *per se*. Many premenopausal women experience swelling, tenderness, some degree of breast discomfort or pain, or increased lumpiness as a result of extra fluid collecting in the breast tissue prior to menstruation. These symptoms usually resolve over time.

Benign breast masses can be divided into three types: (1) nonproliferative—typically a mass with normal cells (e.g., a cyst or fibroadenoma), (2) proliferative without atypia—typically a mass with normal cells but the cells are increasing in number and are otherwise normal, and (3) atypical hyperplasia—cells are increasing in number and do not look normal under a microscope (atypia). Lumps that are characterized as being proliferative without atypia slightly increase the risk of breast cancer, whereas those that are characterized as atypical hyperplasia greatly increase the risk of developing breast cancer.[7]

Common benign breast conditions include fibrocystic changes, fibroadenomas, and breast inflammation. Fibrocystic breast disease, now referred to as fibrocystic breast changes, and fibroadenomas are the most common benign breast conditions that appear as lumps. The following material is adapted from the American Cancer Society.[8]

Fibrocystic Changes

Breast cysts are fluid-filled sacs caused by dilated ducts, and they occur most often in women between ages 20 and 50 and can be found in one or both breasts. Large or small cysts can form when multiplying cells within breast glands and overgrowth of fibers in the supporting tissue cause a blockage in the ducts, thus preventing secretions from draining. The lump may be hard or tender, and some women may experience a sensation of fullness or a dull pain. Many women experience fibrocystic breast changes at some point in their life. Breast changes categorized as fibrocystic are considered normal, and having fibrocystic breasts doesn't increase the risk of breast cancer.

Cysts may come and go, usually presenting before menstruation and subsiding afterward. Having one or more cysts, however, does not necessarily affect one's risk of developing breast cancer. Lumpiness and tenderness fluctuate, especially among premenopausal women, primarily because fibrocystic changes are a response to the levels of ovarian hormones. Some women report that their breast symptoms improve if they avoid caffeine, tea, or chocolate; however, research has not confirmed that eliminating these items from one's diet has a significant impact on symptom relief. Over-the-counter pain relievers, such as acetaminophen (Tylenol, others) or nonsteroidal anti-inflammatory drugs (NSAIDs), such as ibuprofen (Advil, Motrin IB, others), may help relieve the discomfort. Severe pain or large, painful cysts associated with fibrocystic breasts may warrant treatment, including drainage by fine-needle aspiration.

Fibroadenomas

Fibroadenomas are the most common type of benign breast tumor, and most do not increase the risk of breast cancer. They are generally painless, round or oval, firm, and rubbery in consistency; these lumps of the breast tissue arise from an excess growth of glandular and connective tissues. They develop most often during puberty but can occur in women of any age, typically between age 15 and 35. This type of benign tumor can enlarge during pregnancy and breastfeeding and shrink after menopause, as they tend to respond to hormonal changes. They vary in size, and they can enlarge or shrink on their own. A substantial percentage of these lesions may resolve on their own without any treatment.

Fibroadenomas have a typically benign appearance on mammography and can sometimes be diagnosed with fine-needle aspiration or needle core biopsy. Since fibroadenomas can reoccur, it is important to have breast exams at regular intervals.

Hyperplasia (Proliferative Breast Disease)

Hyperplasia, either ductal hyperplasia (also called duct epithelial hyperplasia) or lobular hyperplasia, is an overgrowth of the cells that line the ducts or the milk glands. This condition is described as usual (the cells look very close to normal) or atypical (the cells are more distorted). The latter can be either atypical ductal hyperplasia (ADH) or atypical lobular hyperplasia (ALH). Hyperplasia does not usually cause a lump that can be felt, but it can cause changes that can be seen on a mammogram. It is diagnosed by doing a biopsy.

Unlike other noncancerous breast conditions, hyperplasia, depending on which type, can increase the risk for breast cancer. Mild hyperplasia of the usual type does not increase the risk for breast cancer; however, moderate or florid hyperplasia of the usual type (without atypia) can increase the risk compared to women with no breast abnormalities. The risk of breast cancer among those with atypical hyperplasia (either ADH or ALH) is four to five times higher than that of a woman with no breast abnormalities.

Most types of usual hyperplasia do not require treatment; however, atypical hyperplasia (ADH or ALH), which is found on a needle biopsy, will require further workup to rule out cancer.

Lobular Carcinoma In Situ

Lobular carcinoma in situ (LCIS), not classified as breast cancer despite its name, is a benign growth change in cells lining the lobules of the milk ducts. LCIS does not form a lump or show up on mammography and typically does not spread beyond the lobule. It is diagnosed by needle biopsy. Women diagnosed with LCIS have a 7 to 12 times higher risk of developing invasive cancer in either breast, which indicates that they should be carefully monitored by their physician.

Adenosis

Adenosis, a condition that frequently causes breast pain, occurs when the lobules (milk-producing glands) are enlarged. Mineral deposits (i.e., calcifications) can form in adenosis and show up on mammogram, which is why a biopsy is usually needed to determine if the breast change is caused by adenosis or cancer. That being said, adenosis does not increase the risk of breast cancer.

Fat Necrosis

Fat necrosis is a breast condition that can occur when an area of the fatty breast tissue is damaged, usually as a result of injury to the breast or after breast surgery or radiation treatment. Fat necrosis can form a lump that can be felt, but it is generally painless. Typically, fat necrosis is more common in obese women with very large breasts. This condition does not require treatment and in some instances may go away on its own. It does not increase one's risk of breast cancer.

Intraductal Papillomas

Intraductal papillomas are benign, wart-like tumors that grow within the milk ducts of the breast. Solitary intraductal papillomas, single tumors that often grow in the large milk ducts near the nipple, are a common cause of clear or bloody nipple discharge. Multiple papillomas are seen in small ducts in areas of the breast farther from the nipple and are less likely to cause nipple discharge. Solitary papilloma does not increase the risk of breast cancer (unless it contains other breast changes, such as atypical hyperplasia), but multiple papillomas slightly increase the risk of breast cancer. Surgery is usually performed to remove the papilloma and part of the duct in which it is found.

Nipple Discharge

Secretions or discharge from the nipple are not unusual, but not necessarily a sign of breast disease. Some nipple conditions are related to lactation, while others are not. Premenopausal women, for example, may develop ectasia, a condition when the mammary ducts located under the nipple become dilated (widened). In some cases, ectasia can lead to a blockage of the ducts, causing the fluid to pool and leak into the nearby tissue and cause infection or chronic inflammation. Galactorrhea is a milky discharge from both nipples seen in women who are not breastfeeding. This condition is often due to an increase in the hormone prolactin, which produces milk.

Discharge that occurs when the nipple and breast are squeezed is usually not a cause for concern; however, bloody discharge can indicate a more serious problem that would require medical attention.

Mastitis

Mastitis is an infection most often seen in women who are breastfeeding. Characteristics of mastitis include the breast feeling warm, tender, and lumpy to the touch. The infected part of the breast may appear swollen and red. The cause is usually a blocked milk duct that becomes inflamed and infected if not treated by antibiotics. Warm compresses help alleviate pain, but in some cases, the duct may need to be drained. Mastitis does not raise the risk of developing breast cancer.

Other Benign Breast Conditions

Other benign lumps or tumors that may be found in the breast but are not indicative of breast cancer or do not increase the risk of cancer include lipoma (a fatty tumor), hamartoma (a smooth, painless lump formed by the overgrowth of mature breast cells), hemangioma (a rare tumor made of blood vessels), hematoma (a collection of blood within the breast caused by internal bleeding), adenomyoepithelioma (a very rare tumor formed by certain cells in the milk duct walls), and neurofibroma (a tumor formed by an overgrowth of nerve cells).

Malignant Breast Disease

For most women, being told that she has a suspicious lump in her breast creates a cascade of emotions, with fear topping the list. The immediate thought is that it must be cancer. Cancer refers to a group of diseases in which cells in the body grow, change, and multiply out of control. Thus, breast cancer is a result of erratic, uncontrolled growth and proliferation of cells that originate in the breast tissue. Most breast cancers begin in the ducts that carry milk to the nipple (ductal cancers), and some start in the glands that make breast milk (lobular cancers). A small number of cancers start in other tissues in the breast (e.g., sarcomas and lymphomas). Noninvasive breast cancer refers to cancer cells that are confined to the ducts and do not invade surrounding fatty and connective tissues of the breast. Invasive breast cancer refers to cancer cells that break through the duct and lobular wall and invade the surrounding fatty and connective tissues of the breast.

Breast cancer cells most likely may have been growing for several years before they are able to be detected. If left untreated, there is a significantly greater risk of cancerous cells spreading beyond the breast to other parts of the body via the lymph system.

The lymphatic system plays a central role in the spread of breast cancer, and the axillary (underarm) lymph nodes are particularly important, as they are the first places that cancer cells are likely to be found if the cancer has spread (metastasized). The lymph vessels carry lymph fluid away from the breast. In the case of breast cancer, cancer cells can enter those lymph vessels and start to grow in lymph nodes. The more lymph nodes containing breast cancer cells, the more likely it is that the cancer may be found in parts of the body (metastases). Depending on the location of the tumor, the symptoms may include retraction of the nipple, nipple discharge, and wrinkling or dimpling of the breast skin.

The following describes breast cancer types, the most common being ductal carcinoma in situ, invasive ductal carcinoma, and invasive lobular carcinoma.[9]

Ductal Carcinoma In Situ

Ductal carcinoma in situ (DCIS) of the breast (also called intraductal carcinoma) is an early noninvasive or preinvasive form of breast cancer. A diagnosis of DCIS means that cells that line the milk ducts of the breast are malignant. Symptoms include thickened breast skin, rash or redness on the breast, breast swelling, breast pain, breast dimpling, nipple pain, or an inverted nipple.

DCIS accounts for approximately 20% of all breast cancers, and it is the most common type of noninvasive breast cancer.[10] Generally, in situ tumors are not felt or detected because they are too tiny to have formed a lump, but DCIS can be detected at an early stage by screening mammography. Individuals most at risk for this type of breast cancer include older women (age not well defined, however), women with a history of benign breast disease, women with a family history of breast cancer, and women who do not have children or who are at an older age at the time of the first full-term pregnancy.

The survival rate for DCIS is extremely high, close to 99%. Death related to breast cancer within 10 years after the diagnosis of DCIS occurs in only 1 to 2% of all patients.[11] DCIS usually is treated by lumpectomy followed by radiation therapy. If the DCIS is large, a mastectomy may be recommended. Chemotherapy usually isn't recommended following surgery for DCIS. For those who have surgery, hormone therapy might be considered. If the DCIS is hormone receptor-positive (ER-positive or PR-positive), adjuvant treatment with tamoxifen (for any woman) or an aromatase inhibitor (for women past menopause) for five years after surgery can lower the risk of another DCIS or invasive cancer developing in either breast.[12] Those with recurrent DCIS also have an excellent prognosis, similar to those with early-stage breast cancer.[13] However, DCIS, often described as a noninvasive form of breast cancer, is considered a precursor to, or potential marker for, invasive ductal carcinoma.

Invasive Ductal Carcinoma

Invasive ductal carcinoma (IDC), sometimes called infiltrating ductal carcinoma, accounts for about 80% of all invasive breast cancers in women, the overwhelming majority of whom are over age 55.[14] The symptoms of IDC are similar to those of DICS, and as with DCIS, the cancer originates in the milk ducts. Unlike DCIS, IDC cancer has "invaded" or spread to the surrounding breast tissues. IDC is usually found by mammography and/or ultrasound. Depending on the size and spread of the tumor(s), most women will undergo a combination of any of the following treatments, including surgery (e.g., lumpectomy, mastectomy), radiation therapy, and in some cases hormonal therapy.

In addition to infiltrating ductal carcinoma, there are other more rare subtypes of IDC, including the following.

Medullary Ductal Carcinoma

This tumor is generally small, and the cells are often high grade, which means that they look very different from normal cells and/or are dividing rapidly. Medullary ductal carcinoma can feel like a spongy, soft mass and can be seen on a mammogram. While this cancer can occur at any age, it usually affects women in their late 40s and early 50s, especially in women who have a *BRCA1* mutation. Medullary ductal carcinoma doesn't grow quickly and usually doesn't spread outside the breast to the lymph nodes.[15] It is more responsive to treatment and may have a better prognosis than more common types of invasive ductal cancer. As with any cancer, the treatment plan will depend on the features of the tumor (e.g., type of cells, tumor grade, hormone receptor status, and HER2 status) and the stage of the disease (e.g., tumor size and node status).

Mucinous Ductal Carcinoma

This rare form of invasive ductal cancer, sometimes called colloid carcinoma, is made up of abnormal cells that "float" in pools of mucin, a key ingredient in the slimy, slippery substance known as mucus.[16] This type of breast cancer tends to affect women after they have gone through menopause. Mucinous ductal carcinoma tends to be a less aggressive type that responds well to treatment, has a better prognosis than other types of IDCs, and is less likely to spread to the lymph nodes than other types of breast cancer.

Tubular Ductal Carcinoma

This is another rare type of breast cancer that begins in the milk ducts from which it can spread. Tubular ductal carcinoma tend to be small and grow slowly and are less aggressive than other breast cancers. Women most likely to be diagnosed with this cancer are generally in their early 50s.[17] Tubular breast cancer has an excellent prognosis.

Invasive Papillary Carcinoma

This is the rarest type of IDCs and has a very good prognosis. It begins in the milk ducts and are less likely to involve the lymph nodes. It primarily occurs in women over the age of 60.

Invasive Lobular Carcinoma

Invasive lobular carcinoma (sometimes called infiltrating lobular carcinoma [ILC]) is the second most common type of breast cancer after IDC. Approximately 80% of all invasive breast cancers are invasive ductal carcinomas compared to 10% that are invasive lobular carcinoma.[18] This cancer begins in the milk-producing lobules and spreads to the surrounding breast tissue, and if not found and treated in an early stage, it can spread to the lymph nodes and possibly to other areas of the body. ILC tends to occur later in life than invasive ductal carcinoma—the early 60s as opposed to the mid-to-late 50s. Unlike other invasive breast cancers, ILC tends to be multifocal (there is more than one area of cancer within the breast) and is also more likely to affect both breasts. Symptoms are similar to those for other types of breast cancers; however, ILC is less likely to cause a firm or distinct breast lump. As with other breast cancers, prognosis will depend on whether the cancer has spread, where it has spread, and stage of the disease.

Concluding Thoughts

The preceding discussion reviewed the different types of breast disease, benign and malignant, and described how the female breast has been depicted throughout history. While the female breast has been prominent in art and fashion, information about breast cancer *per se* was largely absent until the 20th century. In fact, breast cancer is not a "new" disease; yet only recently has it been the focus of media attention.

The Edwin Smith Surgical Papyrus, dating to 3000 to 2500 BCE, describes cases of breast cancer, and in the early 400s BCE, Hippocrates, the father of Western medicine, wrote about the physiology and pathology of the breast and the treatment of its diseases, including describing the stages of breast cancer.[19] His description of a diseased breast in a woman more likely than not indicated that she had breast cancer. Centuries later, we now know that there are many types of breast cancer.

In addition to written references to breast cancer, researchers writing in *The Lancet Oncology* found evidence of breast cancer based on their interpretation of Renaissance paintings.[20] Relying on images of the female breast depicted in paintings, they found that two particular Renaissance paintings show females bare breasted whose figures displayed signs of breast cancer. These are believed to be the earliest known depictions of breast cancer in works of art.

The first depiction appears in the painting *The Night* by Michele di Ridolfo del Ghirlandaio (likely painted between 1553 and 1555). In this painting, a nude woman is reclining and sleeping in a dream world, which includes a cherub, an owl, flowers, and various masks. Her left breast is smaller than the right, and her nipple is retracted, all signs of cancer, according to researchers. The second painting, *The Allegory of Fortitude* by Maso da San Friano (1536 to 1571), depicts a female figure sitting on top of a lion. The left breast seems to show swollen tissue around the nipple and an area where a tumor has broken through the skin, typical signs of breast cancer. Though it's hard (if not impossible) to give statistics about the prevalence of cancer at the time, researchers assume that artists would have encountered women with malignant cancers. Proper diagnosis of the disease could not be conclusively made until medicine had the tools and the technology to do so.

Although Scotsman Dr. John Hunter (1728 to 1793) identified lymph as a "cause" of breast cancer, it was not until the late 19th century that breast cancer treatment evolved based on empirical evidence. In 1894, William Halsted published his work on the radical mastectomy based on 50 cases operated at the Johns Hopkins Hospital between 1889 and 1894.[21] Based on his work, the radical mastectomy became the standard surgical procedure used to treat breast cancer well into the 20th century. Based on the work of Marie and Pierre Curie in the late 19th century, radium was used in cancer treatment, and by 1937, radiation therapy was used in addition to surgery to treat breast cancer. Almost 50 years later, researchers showed that women with early-stage breast cancer who were treated with a lumpectomy and radiation have similar survival rates to women treated with only a mastectomy. This will be discussed more fully in subsequent chapters.

Breast diseases are complex, and all cases are not the same. Unlike breast cancers, benign breast conditions are very common and are usually not life threatening. Some, however, are associated with an increased risk of developing breast cancer. Therefore, it is prudent for women to be attuned to changes in the shape, feel, or appearance of their breasts. Any new noticeable change, thickening, or localized swelling/redness in the breast should be brought to the attention of your physician. Aside from a suspicious lump in the breast, other signs of breast disease include a spontaneous clear or bloody discharge from the nipple, retraction or indentation of the nipple, change in the size or contours of the breast, a flattening or indentation of the skin over the breast, and pitting of skin over the breast.

At different times of the month, there can be breast pain, tenderness, and swelling, but these symptoms are probably related to extra fluid that collects in the breast tissue before, during, or after the menstrual period. If, however, any one of these symptoms does not disappear before the next menstrual cycle, a physician should be consulted. There is usually no need to panic, as most of all breast lumps are benign. It is the others that need to be checked out.

Breast changes and warning signs to be aware of include the following:

- Any new lump found in the breast or armpit
- Any lump or thickening that does not shrink or lessen after menstruation

- Any change in the size, shape, or symmetry of the breast(s)
- Any thickening or swelling of the breast(s)
- Any dimpling, puckering, or indentation in the breast(s)
- Any change in the breast skin or nipple
- Any redness or scaliness of the nipple or breast skin
- Any unusual nipple discharge
- Any nipple tenderness or pain that is different from that before or during menstruation

Today, worldwide, breast cancer is the most common cancer in women. That being said, not all women will develop this type of cancer. Who is most at risk in developing breast cancer? What factors contribute to increased risk of developing breast cancer? The next chapter explains the epidemiology of breast cancer as a means of answering these questions.

CHAPTER TWO

Who Is at Risk for Breast Cancer?

Few diseases evoke as much fear as breast cancer. Many women perceive the diagnosis of breast cancer as a devastating life changer, despite the remarkable strides made in breast cancer detection and treatment as well as breast cancer survival. Yes, the diagnosis can be upsetting, but this disease is not uniformly fatal, and there are some very effective treatment options available. The type of treatment naturally will be dictated by many factors, including patient characteristics, type of breast cancer, and hormone receptor status. That being said, today women diagnosed and treated for most types of breast cancer at an early stage have an excellent prognosis for long-term survival.

While most people think of breast cancer as a women's disease (the overwhelming majority of cases are diagnosed in women), men also can develop breast cancer. But breast cancer in men accounts for less than 1% of all breast cancer cases in the United States, and a man's lifetime risk of breast cancer is about 1 in 883 compared to 1 in 8 in women over the course of her lifetime.[1] In 2019, almost 268,600 new cases of invasive breast cancer were diagnosed in American women compared to 2,670 cases in American men.[2] Given that breast cancer is predominantly a "women's disease" and given that population-based screening for breast cancer is done on women, not men, the following will focus only on women.

What Do the Numbers Tell Us?

The American Cancer Society (ACS) and the National Cancer Institute's Surveillance, Epidemiology and End Results (SEER) Cancer Registry, both rich sources of information, compile statistics from which much of the data presented herein is based. Since 1963, the ACS has published its annual Cancer Facts and Figures, which is an excellent source from which to monitor long-term trends in incidence, prevalence, and mortality rates. The SEER program is an epidemiologic surveillance system, consisting of population-based tumor registries designated to track cancer incidence and survival in geographically defined areas in the United States. This registry collects information on all primary cancers, not just breast cancer. Globally, the International Agency for Research on Cancer (IARC), the specialized cancer agency of the World Health Organization (WHO), compiles data to describe the burden of cancer worldwide.

What do the numbers tell us? Approximately 30% of all newly diagnosed cancers in women will be some type of breast cancer.[3] Globally, an estimated 2.1 million women each year are diagnosed with breast cancer. Geographically, breast cancer incidence differs among countries and even within an individual country, with rates higher among women in more developed countries compared to low- and middle-income countries (LMICs). That being said, incidence rates are increasing in nearly every region globally.[4] Regarding mortality, women in LMICs have a much lower survival rate compared to women who live in more developed countries of the world.

In the United States, the number of new cases of noninvasive and invasive breast cancer increased rapidly during the 1980s and 1990s, a primary reason for which is the increase in mammography screening. More women were being screened for breast cancer and more cases were being detected. To a certain extent, the widespread use of mammography served to inflate the incidence rate because cancers were being diagnosed earlier than they would have had screening not been done.[5] This phenomenon will be discussed in the screening chapter in the explanation of lead time and length time bias. Another possible explanation is the decrease in use of hormone therapy that had been routinely used to treat menopausal symptoms. After the publication of a large-scale trial that found a higher risk of breast cancer among those women who were on hormonal therapy, physicians stopped prescribing such medication.[6] The decline was greatest among white women and those 50 years and older probably because this cohort was more likely to be on hormonal therapy compared to other racial/ethnic/age groups.

Over the ensuing decades, breast cancer continues to be the most commonly diagnosed cancer among American women (excluding skin cancer).[7] While the number of newly diagnosed cases of breast cancer has remained somewhat constant, there are some positive trends in the number of breast cancer deaths. Even though breast cancer mortality is higher than that for other cancers (second to lung cancer), deaths from breast cancer overall have decreased substantially over the past decades, although this decrease is more evident in older women compared to younger women (<50 years of age).

Since 2007, breast cancer death rates have been steady in women younger than 50 but have continued to decrease in older women.[8]

The American Cancer Society estimates that currently there are more than 3.5 million breast cancer survivors in the United States, which includes women still being treated and those who have completed treatment. Based on data from the SEER cancer registry, it is estimated that almost 323,000 breast cancer deaths among American women were averted.[9] This decline is attributed to improvements in treatment and early detection.

Who Is at Risk of Developing Breast Cancer?

Whether one develops breast cancer or not depends on many factors. Some women are at higher risk for breast cancer than others, and survival also differs, depending on an individual's genetic, demographic, and clinical factors. The following presentation of the major risk factors associated with breast cancer incidence and survival must be read with the understanding that having one or more risk factors does not automatically imply that an individual will develop breast cancer. All it means is that the risk of breast cancer is higher among those with risk factors compared to those who have no risk factors. It is also important to know that 85% of breast cancers occur in women who have no risk factors.[10]

The concept of risk can be confusing. Basically, a risk factor is something that increases the chance of getting a disease. Smoking, for example, is a risk factor for lung cancer. High cholesterol is a risk factor for heart disease. Some risk factors cannot be changed (e.g., age, ethnicity, genetics), while others relating to behavior can be (e.g., stop smoking, change one's diet). Epidemiology is the science that quantifies not only whether a disease is associated with specific risk factors but also to what extent a specific risk factor increases the odds of developing the disease. This is calculated statistically, allowing for a margin of error, since it is almost impossible to state with statistical certainty that risk factor A causes disease X. That being said, epidemiologists and biostatisticians will look at the strength of association between various risk factors and disease. Is there double the risk of getting the disease? Is there no association between a specific risk factor and the disease? Is there some protective effect? That is, to what extent does a particular factor serve to reduce the odds of the disease developing (e.g., eating broccoli and other cruciferous vegetables has been shown to help prevent colon cancer)?

Epidemiology is a population-based science that relies on data obtained from many individuals (e.g., population groups). While epidemiology can show elevated risk of disease among populations, it cannot specifically state with certainty that one specific individual within that population group will develop a specific disease. The focus of epidemiology is to identify risk factors and determinants of disease among population groups and to apply that information as a means of disease prevention for individuals who may have risk factors that could increase the likelihood of developing the disease. Based on that knowledge, an individual may choose to change one's lifestyle behavior or take more proactive protective action to hopefully remain disease-free. But even doing so may not be sufficient. My mother, for example, was physically active, ate a healthy diet, and did not have a family history of breast cancer; yet she was diagnosed with breast cancer in her early 50s. Determining causation and identifying risks for disease is an inexact science, and uncertainty in findings, even from the most rigorous studies, exists.

Aside from being female, which is the most significant risk factor for developing breast cancer, what other factors increase the risk of breast cancer? Although studies have identified several risk factors as being more compelling or significant for the development of breast cancer, it needs to be stated again that not every woman with one or more of these risk factors will develop the disease, and there will be women with few if any breast cancer risk factors who develop the disease. The following factors have been shown to increase to some degree the chance of developing breast cancer. Women with one or more risk factors might want to have their physician monitor any changes in the breast more closely, as compared to women who do not have any of the risk factors.

Age

Age is one of the most important risk factors for breast cancer, and unlike other potential factors, one cannot do anything to reduce this risk. Aging is an unmodifiable factor! Breast cancer is generally a disease of the older woman, as the majority of cases are diagnosed after age 50. Based on probability statistics, the lifetime risk of a woman being diagnosed with breast cancer in the United States is estimated to be 12%. That is, on average, an individual woman has a 1-in-8 chance of developing breast cancer over an 80-year life span. If one is 20 years old, the odds of developing breast cancer is 1 in 1,732 (e.g., 1 in 1,732 women in this age group can expect to develop breast cancer). If one is 30 years old, the odds are 1 in 228. At age 50, the probability of developing invasive breast cancer in the next 10 years is 1 in 43, and at age 60, the odds are 1 in 29. Clearly, the probability or odds of developing breast cancer increases as one ages.[11] These estimates are based on population averages and, as such, are just that: estimates. An individual's risk may be higher or lower depending on her own personal profile.

Every breast cancer patient/survivor has to cope with her situation in her own way. However, for many reasons, it may be especially more challenging for young women (i.e., younger than age 45) diagnosed with breast cancer.

Although breast cancer is relatively rare in young women—fewer than 5% of all breast cancers diagnosed in the United States occur in women under 40—the numbers are not insignificant.[12] In the United States an estimated 12,150 cases of breast cancer are diagnosed in women under age 40 and approximately 26,393 in women under 45 years of age. Compared to older women, young women diagnosed with breast cancer generally have more aggressive types of breast cancer and poorer survival rates, indicating that breast cancer in younger women differs biologically from that seen in older women.[13] The lowest overall rate of cancer survival are among those aged 25 to 29 years, followed by those aged 20 to 24 years and 30 to 34 years regardless of the subtype of breast cancer.[14]

Young women treated for breast cancer have disproportionately high rates of second malignancies, including contralateral breast cancer (defined as a tumor in the opposite breast that was diagnosed more than six months following the detection of the first cancer). Young breast cancer patients also have unique, different issues to deal with compared to older women with breast cancer. Many issues have to be discussed with their caregivers, including the ability to get pregnant after treatment and potential risks to the fetus if one does get pregnant; how to deal with the possibility of early menopause; how to deal with the impact of treatment on sexual relations; how to deal with raising small children while undergoing treatment; how to deal with concerns about body image after breast cancer-related surgery and treatment; and how to deal with possible psychosocial issues, including anxiety and depression, during and after treatment.

Regardless of age, counseling and managing the breast cancer patient requires a multidisciplinary approach that must take into account not only the clinical management of the treatment but also mental health issues as well as survivorship concerns.[15]

Race/Ethnicity

Race/ethnicity is another unmodifiable risk factor for breast cancer. A large-scale study published in 2003 confirmed what many in the field of oncology suspected. An individual's ethnic background does indeed make a difference in incidence and mortality and is an important factor in breast cancer diagnosis, treatment, and survival.[16] Breast cancer incidence and mortality differ among ethnic groups, as rates are higher among non-Hispanic white (white) and African American women and lowest among Asian/Pacific Islander women. Asian/Pacific Islander women also have the highest rate of survival. In general, breast cancer is diagnosed at an earlier, more localized stage in white women, affording a more favorable prognosis perhaps because of early diagnosis and effective treatment or perhaps because of differences in the histology and aggressiveness of the tumor. African American women are twice as likely as women of other racial and ethnic groups in the United States to be diagnosed with more aggressive types of breast cancer, and African American and Hispanic women tend to have breast cancer diagnosed at a later stage, which leads to a less favorable prognosis. After African American women, the highest mortality is seen in Latinas.

Differences in overall 5-year relative survival rate for breast cancer are also apparent. The 5-year survival rate for breast cancer cases diagnosed between 2008 and 2014 was 81% for African American women compared to 91% for white women. Many plausible explanations could explain this, but it is more than likely that because the cancer was diagnosed at a more advanced stage in African American women, their survival rate is poorer. It could also be that lack of access to health care and the quality of health care received may help explain this disparity. Only 54% of breast cancers in Black women are diagnosed at an early stage, compared to 64% in white women.[17]

Whereas white women over age 45 years have a much higher rate of breast cancer than African American women, the latter tend to have higher incidence rates at younger ages (<age 40) and have a worse prognosis. Younger African Americans have three times the breast cancer mortality of younger white women.[18]

There is considerable controversy as to whether differences in breast cancer diagnosis and survival are attributable to ethnicity or to socioeconomic status (SES) or to some combination thereof. To what extent does SES explain these differences among ethnic groups? SES is strongly correlated with ethnicity, making it difficult to assess whether differences are due to an individual's ethnic background solely, to the individual's economic status solely, or to some combination thereof. There are inherent differences in an individual's lifestyle and diet, which are also influenced by one's SES. To what extent these factors increase the risk of breast cancer within specific ethnic groups needs to be taken into consideration.

An interesting study attempting to disentangle the influence of ethnicity and SES on breast cancer stage, treatment, and survival linked data from the Metropolitan Detroit SEER registry to Michigan Medicaid enrollment files.[19] Before controlling for Medicaid enrollment and poverty, African American women had a higher likelihood than white women of an unfavorable breast cancer outcome. However, after taking into account these factors, the African American women were not different from white women on most outcomes. This finding may imply that ethnicity, *per se*, was not statistically significantly associated with unfavorable breast cancer outcomes; rather, low SES was associated with late-stage breast cancer at diagnosis, type of treatment received, and death. Poverty, low education level, and lack of health insurance, regardless of one's ethnic group, can be powerful factors in outcomes.

Family History/Genetics

You can pick your friends, but you cannot pick your relatives. You are who you are based on your genetic makeup. In the case of breast cancer, family history of breast cancer, especially in a first-degree relative (e.g., grandmother, mother, sister) on your mother or father's side, increases the risk for the disease. Early observations of women who died of breast cancer indicated that these women were more likely than others to have had a family member with breast cancer. These descriptive reports of familial aggregation of breast cancer led to research to help understand the association between genetic risk and breast cancer.

We now know that the risk of breast cancer among women with a family history of the disease with one affected first-degree female relative is two times higher and three to four times higher with more than one affected first-degree female relative compared to women without any family history.[20] If the affected relative was diagnosed younger than age 50, the risk is even greater. A positive family history is a strong risk factor especially for women under the age of 35 years. That being said, the majority of women who have relatives with breast cancer will themselves not develop this cancer. Further, most women who do develop breast cancer actually do not have a family history of the disease. Having a family history is just a risk factor, not an absolute.

With advances in molecular biology, the potential to identify genes that increase the risk of cancers is now possible. There has been a lot of information about two genes in particular that have been shown to increase the risk of breast cancer among those who have inherited mutations in one or both: the *BRCA1* (BReast CAncer gene one) and *BRCA2* (BReast CAncer gene two). Everyone possesses *BRCA1* and *BRCA2* genes, which help regulate cellular growth and suppress the development of tumors; however, mutations to either gene can result in uncontrolled cell growth, which can lead to cancer. Approximately 5 to 10% of breast cancer cases are attributed to *BRCA1* and *BRCA2* mutations, with *BRCA1* mutations being slightly more common than *BRCA2* mutations. However, certain groups have a higher risk than others. For example, Ashkenazi Jewish women are at greater risk of inheriting *BRCA1* and *BRCA2* mutations as compared to other religious/ethnic groups. Also, breast cancer at an early age (younger than age 50) is more likely to be associated with *BRCA1* and *BRCA2* mutations. A study of women with breast cancer diagnosed before age 30 found that half had strong family histories of breast cancer and *BRCA1* and *BRCA2* mutations.[21]

A woman's lifetime risk of developing breast and/or ovarian cancer is greatly increased if she inherits a mutation in *BRCA1* or *BRCA2*. Women with a *BRCA1* mutation have up to a 72% lifetime risk of developing breast cancer, and for those with a *BRCA2* mutation, the lifetime risk is 69%. However, it must be stressed that most breast cancer occurs in the absence of a *BRCA1* or *BRCA2* mutation. Although inheritance of a *BRCA1* or *BRCA2* mutation is an important risk factor for breast cancer, this does not necessarily mean that a woman with *BRCA1* or *BRCA2* mutations will develop the disease. She is at higher risk of doing so. Of course, other factors influence the development of breast cancer, and if these factors could be modified, then the risk could be reduced . . . maybe. There is no guarantee, as was the case with my mother who did not have *BRCA1* or *BRCA2* mutations but still developed breast cancer.

BRCA1 mutations increase the risk of breast, ovarian, pancreatic, cervical, uterine, and colon cancers. *BRCA1* mutations are also associated with an increased risk of triple-negative breast cancer, an aggressive and frequently difficult to treat cancer. More discussion about triple-negative breast cancer will follow in a subsequent section. *BRCA2* mutations increase the risk of breast, ovarian, pancreatic, gallbladder, bile duct, and melanoma cancers.

Mutations in other genes are also associated with breast cancer, but these genetic mutations are much less common than *BRCA1* and *BRCA2* mutations. Other than *BRCA1* and *BRCA2*, there are more than 150 genetic variants that are associated with some degree of risk for breast cancer, but these have not been studied as much as the *BRCA* mutations and will not be discussed.[22] Only two will be briefly mentioned here.

The p53 protein, encoded by the *TP53* tumor suppressor gene, is an inherited mutation associated with an increased risk of developing breast cancer, particularly a more aggressive type of breast disease, and women with p53 mutation have a worse overall survival. p53 plays an important role in suppressing cancer, and with a p53 mutation, the ability to prevent cancer formation is compromised.[23] p53 mutations can also increase the risk of developing other cancers such as leukemia, brain tumors, and cancer of bones or connective tissues. Another gene, *ATM* (ataxia-telangiectasia mutation), helps repair damaged DNA. Inheriting one mutated *ATM* gene has been linked to an increased rate of breast cancer and pancreatic cancer in some families because the mutation stops the cells from repairing damaged DNA.

As more becomes known about genetic changes and the development of breast cancer, more targeted treatments and preventive measures will emerge. But what can one do now to help protect against genetic mutations? Individuals who are at higher risk of developing breast cancer, for example, may opt for genetic testing. Genetic testing through blood tests are available, especially testing for mutations in *BRCA1* and *BRCA2* genes. Also, there are several panel tests available that can identify mutations in several different genes at the same time. However, before genetic testing is done, genetic counseling should be given. One needs to understand what it means to have a genetic mutation and what options are available given this knowledge (e.g., frequent breast cancer screening, different type of breast cancer screening other than mammography). Each individual has to decide whether to get screened or not. This is very much a personal decision to make. There is a trade-off between knowing "too much" and not knowing.

Menstrual Cycles and Endogenous Hormone Levels

Hormones play a major role in the etiology of breast cancer. Estrogen, in particular, is essential for the normal growth and development of the breast. The main forms of estrogen in females (endogenous estrogen) include *estradiol*, the main estrogen made by the ovaries before menopause; *estrone*, a weaker estrogen produced in the ovaries and in fat tissue from other hormones, which is the main estrogen found in women after menopause (although the ovaries continue to produce small amounts of estradiol); and *estriol*, produced almost exclusively during pregnancy. During each menstrual cycle, estrogen and other ovarian hormones signal cells in the breast and uterus to divide and multiply. Cumulative exposure of the breast to estrogen affects the rate of cell division. Since estrogen stimulates cell division, it can increase the chance of making a normal cell into a cancer cell. Approximately 80% of all breast cancers are "ER-positive" (e.g., the cancer cells grow in response to the hormone estrogen) and approximately 65% are also "PR-positive" (e.g., the cancer cells grow in response to progesterone). Breast tumors have estrogen receptors and depend on estrogen for growth. Antiestrogens (such as the drug tamoxifen) can help block the binding of estrogen to its receptor and prevent the hormone from delivering its message to the breast tumor cells to divide and multiply.

The effect of estrogen on breast cancer risk was shown over 100 years ago when researchers found that removing the ovaries of women with breast cancer improved their chances of survival. Women who had their ovaries removed early in life have a very low incidence of breast cancer. It is thought that lifelong exposure to estrogen plays an important role in breast cancer risk. That is, more exposure to estrogen during a woman's lifetime can have an effect on the development of breast cancer.

Early menstruation (younger than age 12) and starting menopause after age 55 have been associated with breast cancer. Studies have shown that breast cancer risk is 20% higher among girls who begin menstruating before age 11 compared to those who begin at age 13 or later. Women who experience menopause at age 55 or older also are at slightly more risk compared to women who begin menopause at a younger age.[24] Having more menstrual cycles exposes a woman to a longer lifetime exposure to the hormones estrogen and progesterone.

Hormone Receptor (HR) and Human Epidermal Growth Factor Receptor-2 (HER2)

The genetic makeup of a breast tumor enables pathologists to determine the type of cancer and help guide decisions about which treatments are best. Hormonal-receptor positive (HR+) and hormonal-receptor negative (HR–) breast cancer will dictate the nature of the treatment options. Both HR+ and HR– and HER2 in a breast cancer tumor define the most common types of breast cancer. When breast cancer cells have too much of the HER2 protein, the cells grow and divide too quickly. HER2 can either be positive or absent/ negative in the tumor.[25]

One could be HR+ and test positive for the HER2 protein (e.g., HR+ and HER2+). Approximately one in five breast cancers are HER2+, and this type of breast cancer tends to be more aggressive than other types of breast cancer, but treatments that specifically target HER2 have been shown to be effective. Additionally, one could be HR– and HER2+, and in this case, the tumors tend to be more aggressive.

HR–/HER2+ is usually treated with multiple types of treatment, including chemotherapy and targeted HER2+ treatments, but not hormonal therapies.

HR+ and HER2 negative (HER2–) breast cancer is the most common form of breast cancer, accounting for more than 70% of all breast cancers. Another type of breast cancer is triple-negative breast cancer (TNBC). In such cases, one tests negative for estrogen receptors, progesterone receptors, and excess HER2 protein. These results mean the growth of the cancer is not fueled by the hormones estrogen and progesterone, or by the HER2 protein. As such, triple-negative breast cancer does not respond to hormonal therapy medicines or medicines that target HER2 protein receptors. About 15 to 20% of all breast cancers are TNBC. TNBC is more frequently found among younger women, African American women, and women who have *BRCA1* mutation.[26] Triple-negative tumors can be aggressive and have a poorer survival rate than other types of tumors, primarily because at this point in time there are fewer targeted medicines that can effectively treat triple-negative breast cancer.

Hormone Replacement Therapy (HRT)

During menopause, a woman's body undergoes a huge change, including a drop in estrogen. Hormone replacement therapy (HRT) had been prescribed to help alleviate the symptoms of menopause. Millions of prescriptions were written to help replace the body's lost estrogen. However, it became apparent that there were serious risks associated with taking HRT, including higher risk of heart attack, stroke, blood clots, and breast cancer. The Women's Health Initiative (WHI) large-scale, multicenter randomized clinical trial provided conclusive evidence that the harms of taking HRT outweighed the potential benefits, and the Federal Drug Administration (FDA) strongly advised physicians to stop prescribing HRT to menopausal patients because of the serious risks associated with taking this medication.

The WHI showed that not only did HRT increase the incidence of breast cancer, but these tumors were diagnosed at a more advanced stage. HRT apparently stimulated breast cancer growth and density of breast tissue, making breast cancer diagnosis more difficult and increasing the possibility that the cancer would be diagnosed at a more advanced stage, a terrible combination of increasing the risk of disease while also delaying its detection. The clinical trial showed that use of combined estrogen and progestin HRT was harmful to otherwise healthy women.

Use of Oral Contraceptives

Because hormonal factors are known to influence the development of breast cancer and because oral contraceptives (OCs) work by manipulating hormones, there has been concern that taking OCs could increase the risk of breast cancer. Over 80% of American women born since 1945 have used some type of OC at some point in their life. Many epidemiological studies have investigated whether hormonal contraceptives affect breast cancer risk and to what extent is the risk elevated. Based on the evidence, use of OCs (combined estrogen and progesterone) is associated with a small increase in breast cancer risk, particularly among women who begin its use before age 20 or before their first pregnancy.[27] However, this risk diminishes when women stop taking the pill, and after 10 years of not taking OCs, the risk is similar to those who had never taken OCs. It should be noted that early generation OC pills had high-dose estrogen formulations while newer low-dose estrogen formulations may not increase the risk as much, if at all.

Use of injectable progestin-only contraceptive (e.g., Depo-Provera) does not appear to be associated with an increased risk of breast cancer, nor does the levonorgestrel-releasing intrauterine device (e.g., Mirena) appear to increase the risk. Based on available evidence, the overall cancer risk is low, and if an individual had used these contraceptives, any elevation in risk is temporary.

Diethylstilbestrol (DES)

The estrogen synthetic diethylstilbestrol (DES) was prescribed to millions of pregnant women in the United States, particularly in the 1940s through 1971, to prevent miscarriage, premature labor, and related complications of pregnancy. In 1971, researchers linked prenatal DES exposure to a type of cancer of the cervix and vagina (clear cell adenocarcinoma) in a small group of women.[28] Publication of this study caused the drug to be taken off the American market, although the drug continued to be prescribed to pregnant women in Europe until 1978.

DES's relationship to the development of breast cancer in daughters has been studied over the years. The thinking was that DES exposure may increase the growth of any cells that develop into breast cancer and that the daughters would be at greater risk of developing breast cancer compared to women whose mothers did not take DES. While the research is not conclusive, it appears that DES daughters under age 40 did not have a higher risk while DES daughters over age 40 were 2.5 times more likely to develop breast cancer.[29] Caution in interpreting this finding is warranted because the median age of the study group was 43 years old and the women had not yet reached the prime age when breast cancer would be more likely to be diagnosed. While a European study found no elevated risk,[30] a 2011 U.S. study found that about 2% of a large cohort of DES daughters has developed breast cancer due to their exposure.[31]

In Vitro Fertilization (IVF)

Since the drugs used for ovulation induction as part of in vitro fertilization (IVF) treatment increase the levels of endogenous gonadal hormones, there are legitimate concerns about increasing the risk of breast cancer. A systematic review of studies looking at the relationship of IVF and the development of breast cancer found that overall, there is no clear evidence that ovulation induction or IVF increases the risk of breast cancer.[32] Since many women who had IVF have not yet reached the age at which breast cancer would be more likely to develop, we just do not know the extent to which IVF would increase the risk.

On a slightly more positive, encouraging note, a large long-term study of Dutch women who had fertility treatment in the Netherlands between 1980 and 1995 found that IVF treatment compared with non-IVF treatment was not associated with increased risk of breast cancer after a median follow-up of 21 years. Breast cancer risk among IVF-treated women was also not significantly different from that in the general population.[33]

More research needs to be done in order to answer the following questions: What are the long-term effects of ovulation-stimulating drugs? How many treatment cycles would increase the risk of breast cancer? To what extent does having IVF in one's 20s increase the risk as opposed to having IVF in one's 30s? To what extent does having a family history of breast cancer increase the risk of breast cancer after IVF?

Lifestyle Factors

As with other types of disease, there is an association between various lifestyle risk factors and developing breast cancer. Unlike some of the unmodified risk factors discussed above, there are many other factors that can be modified, which may help reduce breast cancer risk. Trying to tease out which factors are "more important" than others, however, is difficult since many lifestyle factors are intertwined. This situation is often the case in chronic diseases, as there are many factors, for example, that influence the development of heart disease. There is no "one factor" that if eliminated would prevent heart disease. The same is true for cancer. However, working to reduce modifiable risk factors can have a positive effect, all things considered. The following is a short list of modifiable risk factors for breast cancer.

Overweight, obesity, and body mass are known risk factors for breast cancer that have been documented in numerous studies. Fat tissue is the largest source of estrogen in postmenopausal women, and higher amounts of estrogen in the blood are linked to an increased risk of breast cancer in women after menopause. But there is a twist because it depends on at what point in one's life that one is overweight/obese. The research shows that while overweight women have a lower risk of breast cancer before menopause, there is a higher risk after menopause. Many studies have shown that adult weight gain and body fatness and distribution (e.g., a body mass index (BMI) above 25 kg/m^2 and abdominal fatness) are associated with an *increased risk of postmenopausal* breast cancer.[34] Greater body fatness during childhood and adolescence, however, is associated with *reduced risk of premenopausal* breast cancer, independent of adult BMI and menstrual cycle characteristics.[35] One possible explanation is that overweight or obesity in premenopausal women may reduce exposure to ovarian hormones. In contrast, overweight or obesity in postmenopausal women may increase estrogen levels, leading to an increase in breast cancer risk.[36]

Women who gain a lot of weight over the decades have almost twice the risk of breast cancer compared to women who tend to keep their weight steady. Each 5 kg (about 11 pounds) that one gains during adulthood increases the risk of postmenopausal breast cancer by 11%.[37] Yet this risk does not seem to be as great for those who have been overweight since childhood. The relationship between overweight, obesity, and BMI to breast cancer risk is complex, but the available evidence seems to indicate that if one can keep one's weight within the ranges of a normal BMI (18.5 to 25 kg/m^2), the risk for postmenopausal breast cancer is reduced. Certainly there are other factors that must be taken into account, including diet, for example.

Many studies have looked at the role of *diet* in breast cancer development. A Mediterranean diet consisting of vegetables, fruits, whole grains, fish, and olive oil has consistently been associated with a decreased risk of not only heart disease but also breast cancer.[38] There is also some evidence that a diet rich in high in dietary fiber may be protective as well. Conversely, studies show that high-fat diets, particularly those rich in red meat consumption, have been linked to higher risk of breast cancer. A systematic review of studies that investigated the link between the consumption of red and processed meats and breast cancer incidence concluded that eating processed meats is statistically associated with an increased risk for breast cancer, and eating white meat (e.g., poultry) confers a reduced risk.[39] The researchers concluded that if women ate less red meat and less processed meats their risk for breast cancer would be reduced. Over 42,000 women were followed for an average of seven and a half years. Previous studies had found inconsistent results, but this large-scale review show a clear statistical assòciation between consumption of red meat and breast cancer. It should be noted that diet studies are notorious difficult to conduct, and it is very difficult to separate the effects of diet from other factors.

Alcohol consumption is also a potential factor in contributing to many diseases, but there are so many different alcoholic beverages, and people metabolize alcohol differently, making it very difficult to pinpoint exactly alcohol's effect on breast cancer development. In all probability, alcohol consumption has some effect, which is why it is recommended that individuals avoid excessive alcohol consumption. But how one defines "excessive" is another problematic issue.

Tobacco smoking is well known to be carcinogenic, not only for breast cancer but also for most types of cancer. Many large-scale studies published over the past decade show a positive association between tobacco smoking and breast cancer. The 2014 report of the U.S. Surgeon General estimates a 10% increase in breast cancer risk for women with a history of smoking,[40] and the American Cancer Society's Cancer Prevention Study II (CPS-II) Nutrition Cohort further supports the carcinogenic effect of smoking.[41] Women who started smoking before the birth of their first child had a higher risk of breast cancer than women who never smoked. The study also found a higher incidence of breast cancer in long-term, heavy-smoking current and former smokers than in people who had never smoked.

Physical activity, or lack thereof, has been associated with numerous diseases, including cancer. Findings from a large prospective cohort study analyzing almost 74,000 postmenopausal women found a 25% lower risk for breast cancer in the most physically active group compared to the least physically active group. Walking seems to be the most frequent type of physical activity that people engage in.[42] Findings from the large-scale Women's Health Initiative (WHI) study (from 1993 to 1998) provide encouraging results about the potential benefits of exercise. Compared with less active women, women who engaged in 1.25 to 2.5 hours a week of brisk walking had an 18% decreased risk of breast cancer. A slightly greater reduction in risk was seen for women who engaged in the equivalent of 10 hours or more per week of brisk walking. Those who exercised for longer periods of time and engaged in more strenuous activity showed the most benefit.

The take-home message about physical activity is that exercise need not be vigorous in order to confer a health benefit. Whether one spends hours in the fitness club each week doing aerobic exercises or takes several brisk walks a week, there is a positive potential benefit to the activity. Exercising daily or a few times a week not only can help reduce the risk of breast cancer but can also result in weight loss and improvements in cardiovascular fitness. Regular physical activity can not only help maintain a healthy body weight but also cause positive changes in a women's metabolism or immune factors, which could help protect against breast cancer.

While there is strong evidence that being physically active at all ages is protective against breast cancer, there are many unanswered questions, including what type of exercise, intensity level, duration of the physical activity, and so forth confer the "best" protection against disease. In the meantime, staying active, even if walking 30 minutes a day, can't hurt and probably can be helpful in staying healthy.

Pregnancy and Breast Cancer

In the early 18th century, Bernardino Ramazzini, an Italian physician whose notable contribution to medicine was in identifying occupational diseases, noted a higher frequency of breast cancer among nuns than in married women. Centuries later, epidemiological studies confirmed that nuns and those who never had children had higher rates of breast cancer, most probably because they do not benefit from the protective effect of having children and breastfeeding. Evidence shows that a woman has a 7% decreased risk of breast cancer per birth, and her risk drops by an additional 4% for every year of breastfeeding.[43]

Being pregnant when breast cancer is diagnosed complicates things greatly, and the prognosis is not favorable. However, getting pregnant and giving birth after a diagnosis of breast cancer does not increase mortality. Breast surgery can be done in all trimesters of pregnancy, but radiation therapy is not recommended until after delivery of the baby to avoid radiation exposure to the fetus. Chemotherapy, however, can be given safely during pregnancy in the second and third trimester. Naturally, breast cancer survivors should discuss the pros and cons of getting pregnant with their physician. Issues of fertility preservation and embryo cryopreservation should be explored as well. There are options!

Breast Characteristics

Evidence suggests a relationship between breast tissue characteristics, especially breast density, and increased risk of breast cancer. Breast tissue is composed of milk glands, milk ducts and supportive tissue (dense breast tissue), and fatty tissue (non-dense breast tissue). Breast tissue density is a mammographic indicator of the amount of glandular and connective tissue relative to fatty tissue. When viewed on a mammogram, women with dense breasts have more dense tissue than fatty tissue. Fat appears as radiologically lucent areas, whereas connective and epithelial tissue appear as areas of high radiologic density. On a mammogram, non-dense breast tissue appears dark and transparent. Conversely, dense breast tissue appears as a solid white area on a mammogram, which makes it much more difficult to interpret and could mask possible breast tumors. Dense breast tissue cannot be felt in a clinical breast exam or in a breast self-exam.

It is estimated that nearly half of all women aged 40 and older have some degree of breast density as found on mammogram. Women who are younger, have a low body mass index, or take hormone therapy for menopause are more likely to have dense breasts. In general, breast density decreases with age, pregnancy, menopause, and higher body weight. There are several levels of breast density, including almost entirely fatty (e.g., the breasts are almost entirely composed of fat), scattered areas of fibroglandular density (e.g., there are some scattered areas of density, but the majority of the breast tissue is non-dense), heterogeneously dense (e.g., there are some areas of non-dense tissue, but the majority of the breast tissue is dense), and extremely dense (e.g., nearly all of the breast tissue is dense). Women with very dense breasts have the highest risk that cancer would not be detected on a film mammogram, and other screening modalities should be considered (e.g., digital mammogram or MRI of the breast). This will be discussed in more detail in another chapter.

Women with denser breasts (containing more connective and glandular tissue) have been shown to be at higher risk for breast cancer. Women with breasts that are less dense (e.g., containing more fatty tissue) appear to be a lesser risk, perhaps because less dense breasts are easier to interpret on mammogram. As of December 2018, more than 70% of U.S. states have passed laws requiring that mammography reports include information about breast density and that women be notified of their breast density with mammography results.[44]

Other breast characteristics can increase the risk of breast cancer, including benign breast conditions that represent a spectrum of disorders.[45] For example, *nonproliferative lesions* (e.g., fibrocystic changes, fibrocystic disease, chronic cystic mastitis, and mammary dysplasia), the most common of which are breast cysts, are associated with little to no increased breast cancer risk. *Proliferative lesions without atypia* (e.g., ductal hyperplasia without atypia, intraductal papillomas, sclerosing adenosis, radial scars, and fibroadenomas) are associated with a small increased risk of developing breast cancer. *Proliferative lesions with atypia* (e.g., atypical ductal hyperplasia and atypical lobular hyperplasia) are associated with the greatest risk of developing breast cancer. These lesions have some, but not all, of the features of ductal carcinoma in situ (DCIS) or lobular carcinoma in situ (LCIS).

Other benign breast disorders, including lipoma (usually solitary tumors composed of mature fat cells), fat necrosis of the breast (most commonly occurs as the result of breast trauma or surgery), and adenomas (epithelial neoplasms of the breast) do not increase the risk of breast cancer.

Do breast implants increase the risk of breast cancer? Until recently, the consensus was that there is no association between breast implants and risk of breast cancer. That being said, breast implants can obstruct the view of breast tissue, which is why women with implants should tell the mammography technician about their implants and probably arrange to have more complete breast imaging scheduled. Recently, there is evidence that women with a particular type of implant are at increased risk for a rare type of lymphoma, anaplastic large cell lymphoma (BIA-ALCL), a rare cancer of the immune system.[46] It is not breast cancer *per se*, but the cancer develops in tissue around the implant. The main symptoms of the lymphoma include swelling and fluid accumulation around the implant. Specifically, the textured breast implants made by Allergan have been linked to this rare cancer, and the Food and Drug Administration (FDA) recalled the implant as of July 24, 2019. The FDA's decision was based on an uptick in the number of cases and deaths from implant-associated cancer. Interestingly, the Allergan devices were banned in Europe in late 2018.

Breastfeeding

Breastfeeding is thought to be a protective factor in the development of breast cancer, primarily because of the hormonal changes it confers, especially a decrease in the level of estrogen. As such, a women's risk of developing breast cancer would be reduced as a result of lower estrogen levels. Women who breastfeed experience hormonal changes during lactation that delay their menstrual periods, which could affect the number of ovulatory cycles a woman would have over the course of her reproductive lifetime. The less one ovulates, the less the exposure to estrogen and abnormal cells that could become cancer. The potential positive impact that breastfeeding has was empirically studied by the Collaborative Group on Hormonal Factors in Breast Cancer. This large, multinational study compared mothers who breastfed to those who did not, and the findings showed that for every 12 months a woman breastfed, the risk of breast cancer decreased by 4.3%.[47]

Breastfeeding also may cause physical changes in the cells that line the mammary ducts, which may make the cells more resistant to mutations that could lead to cancer. However, it is difficult to say with certainty whether it is the breastfeeding that confers protection or is a combination of other factors.

Environmental Exposures

Environmental factors have been thought to contribute to the development of breast cancer. Probably the most comprehensive study to assess environmental/chemical exposure and the relationship to breast cancer is the Long Island Breast Cancer Study Project, one of the largest studies ever conducted on the environmental causes of breast cancer.[48] The purpose of this large study was to investigate the high rate of breast cancer in Long Island, New York. The study focused on exposure to specific pollutants, including organochlorine pesticides, including DDT and its metabolite DDE; polychlorinated biphenyls (PCBs); toxic compounds used in electrical transformers; and polycyclic aromatic hydrocarbons (PAHs), a primary component of urban air pollution. Environmental samples of water and soil were tested for pesticides and metals.

After careful analysis, the findings did not show a clear link between breast cancer and exposure to environmental pollutants. Although there was some evidence of a modest increase in the risk of breast cancer from PAH exposure, the researchers did not identify any environmental factors that could be responsible for the high incidence of breast cancer in the Long Island area. Another study failed to show an association between exposure to electromagnetic fields from residential power use and breast cancer risk.[49]

A large study is currently underway to identify the interplay between genetics and the environment. The Sister Study, funded by the federal government, recruited more than 50,000 women who are sisters. The study will compare the genetic profiles and environmental exposures of sisters who did not develop breast cancer with those who did. Early findings show that women who lived in areas of higher airborne lead, mercury, and cadmium were at a higher risk of developing postmenopausal breast cancer; that young women with high body fat have a decreased chance of developing breast cancer before menopause; and that high levels of vitamin D in the blood, and regular vitamin D supplement use, were associated with lower rates of postmenopausal breast cancer.[50]

Radiation Exposure

Radiation exposure is ubiquitous, coming from many different sources some of which are natural and others man-made. The earth's crust is a major source natural radiation, with natural deposits of uranium, potassium, and thorium accounting for the release of small amounts of ionizing radiation. Ionizing radiation in large doses can damage cells, causing them to mutate in ways that may eventually lead to cancer. Airborne radon, a radioactive gas that emanates from the ground, is also a major source of radiation.

On average, Americans receive a radiation dose of about 0.62 rem (620 millirem) each year, with half of this dose originating from natural background radiation (e.g., radon in the air). The good news is that in general, a yearly dose of 620 millirem from all radiation sources has not been shown to cause humans any harm. But by far, the most significant source of man-made radiation exposure is from medical procedures, such as diagnostic x-rays, nuclear medicine, and radiation therapy. In general, the more radiation a person is exposed to and the younger the age at exposure, the greater the risk of developing cancer.

Exposure to radiation sources has been linked to many cancers, including most types of leukemia (although not chronic lymphocytic leukemia); multiple myeloma; and thyroid, bladder, lung, ovarian, and colon (but not rectal) cancers. Breast cancer, too, may also develop from radiation exposure. Exposure to ionizing radiation during childhood and adolescence, for example, increases the risk for breast cancer later in life. Very low doses of radiation (such as from x-rays), however, do not have much, if any, impact on breast cancer risk, although high-dose radiation therapy logically confers a much higher risk of cancer.

Some women fear that having a mammogram will increase the risk of cancer. Although the radiation during mammography can increase the risk of breast cancer over time, this increase is very small.[51,52] Further, when evaluating radiation-induced breast cancer risk, it is important to consider variation in radiation dose from a single examination. Exams vary in the number of views performed and dose per view. Radiation dose is strongly correlated with compressed breast thickness; thus, large-breasted women tend to receive higher doses per view and may require more than four views for complete examination.[53] Women with large breasts can be exposed to 1.8 times higher radiation dose, on average, than women without large breasts.[54] Additionally, age at first mammogram (e.g., age 45 vs. age 50) and screening frequency will also affect the odds of radiation-induced breast cancer. Prior medical history also will have an impact. The risk of breast cancer is higher for women treated with radiation therapy to the chest area before age 20, but is very small for a woman treated after age 40.

If one is weighing the pros and cons of having a mammogram, it is important to know that studies show the benefits of screening mammography outweigh the risk from radiation exposure, especially for women aged 50 and older. Further, radiation treatments have evolved and now include lower doses given over smaller targeted areas. The following chapter goes into much more detail about the potential harm from radiation exposure.

Factors That Are Not Associated with Breast Cancer Risk

The belief that having an abortion will increase the risk of breast cancer is false. There are numerous studies that have looked at the relationship and found no link between breast cancer and abortion (either spontaneous or induced). There also is no empirical relationship between use of hair dyes or hair relaxers with breast cancer. Exposure to electromagnetic fields (from utility wires, electric blankets, etc.) and cell phones does not increase the risk of breast cancer. Deodorant/antiperspirant use is not associated with breast cancer. Caffeine and sugar do not increase the risk of breast cancer, nor does previous breast trauma. Taking antidepressants will not increase the risk of breast cancer. Suffice it to say, research has shown which factors increase the risk of breast cancer, which should help in the understanding of how this cancer develops.

Concluding Thoughts

While many factors *may* contribute to the development of breast cancer, and I stress may, the likelihood of getting breast cancer is complex and at times perplexing. My mother could not understand why or how she got breast cancer since in her mind, she "did everything right" to prevent cancer. In her case, she was of a prime age for breast cancer to develop (mid-50s), she was an Ashkenazi Jew, and her mother died of stomach cancer (which may or may not have anything to do with my mother's breast cancer). She also did not have a mammogram, and by the time her breast cancer was diagnosed, it had metastasized to several lymph nodes.

Today, there are many screening tests that enable physicians to screen for breast disease. While the mammogram is probably the most commonly used population-based screening test, over the past decade there have been many advances in breast cancer detection. Depending on one's risk of breast cancer, one or more of the screening tests might be recommended. The following chapters review these options.

CHAPTER THREE

Screening for Disease: The Pros and Cons

How many times have we heard, or even said to ourselves, "An ounce of prevention is worth a pound of cure"? We might say this when thinking about purchasing insurance for a home or car or installing hurricane shutters to limit damage from heavy rain and wind to one's home or place of business. The quote is ascribed to Benjamin Franklin who, after visiting Boston and seeing how they handled fires, wrote an anonymous letter advocating fire prevention to the City of Philadelphia in 1736. Presumably his reasoning was that preventing a fire would be less costly than dealing with the consequences of the fire. The implication is that it is preferable to be proactive rather than to react to a problem after the fact.

When dealing with one's health, most people would prefer to be proactive rather than reactive. Wouldn't preventing disease be better than dealing with the disease once it develops? Shouldn't health care be a "right" for all in order to prevent serious disease from causing undo harm and even death? The U.S. Declaration of Independence contains the phrase "life, liberty and the pursuit of happiness," which are stated explicitly as unalienable rights as conceived by the authors of the document. Health, however, is not mentioned as an unalienable right. The U.S. Constitution does not set forth an explicit right to health care, and the Supreme Court has never interpreted the Constitution as guaranteeing a right to health care services from the government.

The U.S. Congress continues to vigorously debate this issue with proponents making the case that health care should be recognized as a human right and opponents arguing, among other things, that health care is a service that should be paid for; it is not considered a right *per se*. But if Franklin's quote is taken literally and applied to illness and disease, wouldn't providing services and programs to identify disease at an early stage, before it progresses to a more advanced and presumably more serious stage, save lives and enable individuals to enjoy a healthy, hopefully disease-free life?

Preventive health care, a universal staple in almost all health care systems in the developed world, is designed to promote *disease prevention*, as opposed to *disease treatment*. Seeing your doctor for routine checkups, having a healthy and balanced lifestyle, and staying up to date with immunizations are just some ways to prevent disease or, more accurately, promote good health. Screening for disease is another important component of preventive health care. In terms of diseases and conditions that often show no warning signs (e.g., high blood pressure), preventive health screenings can be very effective at showing early disease risk so that proactive steps can be taken to prevent chronic illnesses from becoming a serious medical issue, including death.

Does Screening Save Lives?

Does screening save lives? In actuality, the answer is not always simple, and findings from the clinical trials that form the basis for validating a screening test are not always in agreement. Also, the answer to the question will depend on the specific disease to be screened and the reliability and accuracy of the screening test to be used. Most of the common screening tests used are not 100% accurate. Sometimes people without the disease test positive, and sometimes those with the disease test negative. More on this later.

It is important to understand that a screening test is designed to identify those who *may* have a disease. A basic tenet of screening is that people getting screened are presumed to be disease-free at the time of the screening. These individuals may appear to be healthy with no signs or symptoms or may unknowingly be presymptomatic. The point is we don't know who may have the disease at the time of screening. The objective of the screening test is not to identify people who already have been diagnosed with disease X and then do a screening test. That is not what screening is designed to do. The test is designed to identify individuals who *might be at risk* of developing a specific disease prior to clinical presentation, and these individuals would then be referred for further testing in order to rule in or rule out disease.

A Short History of Population-Based Screening

Population-based screening for disease is not a new concept. Screening for psychiatric disorders in the U.S. Army is probably the oldest screening program in the United States. The U.S. military developed methods to rapidly screen the mental health of World War I and II draftees, which were designed to exclude recruits with psychological disorders from joining the army.[1]

Intelligence testing and a brief psychological screening test were included as part of the physical exam at the time. Currently, only three mental health tools are used to screen applicants before their entrance into military service: educational achievement (e.g., graduation from high school), cognitive testing, and a cursory psychiatric evaluation.

In the early 20th century, screening for infectious diseases such as tuberculosis (TB), gonorrhea, and syphilis was instituted[2] and found to be extremely valuable as a public health preventive measure and as a model to prevent the spread of disease in the population. In 1936, Thomas Parran, the U.S. Surgeon General, established a program for controlling syphilis that included mandatory premarital and prenatal blood tests. Whether the test had been done prenatally, and if the test was not done an explanation as to why not, had to be so noted on the birth certificate. Women and physicians could refuse on religious or other grounds. By 2001, 46 states and the District of Columbia had laws regarding antenatal syphilis screening. Thirty-four states mandate one prenatal test, usually at the first prenatal visit or early in pregnancy, and 12 include third-trimester testing for all or high-risk women.[3]

Screening for other infectious diseases such as HIV and hepatitis B and C is also valuable at the individual level as well as at the societal level.[4] Individuals who test positive on screening are referred to a health care provider for confirmatory diagnosis and appropriate treatment, which hopefully would serve to limit the spread of the disease in the general population.

Screening for chronic diseases such as hypertension, high cholesterol, and diabetes can identify people who are at risk of developing disease based on the results of a screening test. Those with abnormal test results are referred to affirm the presence of the disease and then receive appropriate treatment. The logic is that early detection and subsequent intervention could save lives by initiating treatment before the disease progresses to a more serious level.

One of the first population-based, large-scale community screening programs for chronic disease focused on screening for diabetes, which was conducted in 1946 to 1947 in Oxford, Massachusetts, by the U.S. Public Health Service. Diabetes, then and now, is underdiagnosed, and compounding the problem is that most people with diabetes do not even know that they have the condition until years after onset. In 1953, tablets for testing urine glucose become widely available, and in 1964, the first strips for testing blood glucose were introduced. Today many tests are used to screen for and diagnose diabetes, including the hemoglobin A1C, fasting blood glucose, and the oral glucose tolerance tests.

In the 1950s, the term "multiphasic screening" was first applied to a health survey in San Jose, California. The multiphasic survey was conceived with a view to combining several of screening tests in one "package" rather than screening for single diseases.[5]

A simple uniform record was used, and in some instances a short history form was also provided, covering questions that related to symptoms that might indicate heart disease, tuberculosis, syphilis, diabetes, rheumatism, defects of eyesight or hearing, or other disabilities.

In the early 1960s, newborn screening programs in the United States began thanks to the work of Dr. Robert Guthrie who developed a screening test for phenylketonuria (PKU), a hereditary metabolic disorder and the first disorder for which newborns were routinely screened.[6] Newborn screening is an important means of identifying disorders that if not diagnosed and treated at an early stage can negatively impact long-term health. Early detection, diagnosis, and treatment of certain genetic, metabolic, or infectious congenital disorders can lead to significant reductions of death, disease, and associated disabilities. Newborn screening has expanded since the introduction of PKU testing, and today approximately 54 conditions are now routinely screened for in newborns in the United States.

The development of a cervical cancer cytological test, the Papanicolaou ("Pap") smear, is perhaps one of the greatest achievements of population-based screening. The test, developed by Dr. George Papanicolaou in the 1940s, detects the cancerous cells in their preclinical phase, affording an excellent prognosis as a result of early diagnosis and treatment. The number of women dying from cervical cancer in the United States declined dramatically after the Pap test was integrated into the gynecologic exam.

Mass screening of breast cancer started when mammography became available as a screening test in the 1960s and will be discussed in depth in subsequent chapters specific to cancer screening.

In summary, disease screening has become one of the most basic tools of modern public health and preventive medicine. Pregnant women are routinely tested for many conditions. Newborns, as previously discussed, are routinely tested for metabolic and neural tube abnormalities. Blood pressure, diabetes, glaucoma, and other diseases are routinely screened for. Many states, but not all, have initiated mandatory screening for sickle cell disease, focusing on population groups that are at high risk for this disease (e.g., African Americans).

As the concept of population-based screening gained acceptance in both the lay and medical communities, it became apparent that criteria to evaluate screening programs were lacking. There were no guidelines focusing on the appropriateness of a specific screening test, at what point during the lifespan individuals should be screened, who should be screened, and even which diseases should be screened. In 1961, Thorner and Remein of the U.S. Public Health Service published a monograph, *Principles and Procedures in the Evaluation of Screening for Disease*, which was the first comprehensive review to set forth the principles of screening.[7] In 1968, the World Health Organization published a monograph by Wilson and Jungner, *The Principles and Practice of Screening for Disease*.[8] The Wilson and Jungner monograph, in particular, proposed 10 "principles" for evaluation of screening program, which are still considered to be highly relevant. In fact, the WHO considers it to be a public health classic.

Wilson and Jungner Classic Screening Criteria

1. The condition sought should be an important health problem.
2. There should be an accepted treatment for patients with recognized disease.
3. Facilities for diagnosis and treatment should be available.
4. There should be a recognizable latent or early symptomatic stage.
5. There should be a suitable test or examination.
6. The test should be acceptable to the population.
7. The natural history of the condition, including development from latent to declared disease, should be adequately understood.
8. There should be an agreed policy on whom to treat as patients.
9. The cost of case-finding (including diagnosis and treatment of patients diagnosed) should be economically balanced in relation to possible expenditure on medical care as a whole.
10. Case-finding should be a continuing process and not a "once and for all" project.

Based on these 10 tenets, a screening program should begin with the goal of reducing an adverse health outcome in a specific population, and there should be a measurable benefit of earlier treatment (e.g., after screening detection) versus later treatment (e.g., after clinical detection).[9] Potential harms include overdiagnosis, false positive and false negative results, and these concepts will be discussed further in another section. The key issue in making a decision to initiate a population-based screening program or not is: would early detection, as compared with later detection, lead to an increase in disease identification and early treatment with the potential for reducing potentially adverse effects on health? Thus, when thinking about introducing a screening program, it is very important to assess the magnitude of potential health benefits as compared to the magnitude of potential health harms in order to determine net benefits of a specific disease screening test. This "balance approach" to screening relies on data and should be continually reassessed as new information is accumulated. Screening can be a "double-edged sword." It can lead to either net benefits or net harms. The trick is to minimize the harms.

In the 1970s, Canada and the United States embraced population-based screening and established governmental agencies to promote screening programs: the Canadian Task Force on the Periodic Health Examination and the U.S. Preventive Services Task Force (USPSTF). Each serves to evaluate the relevance and importance of specific screening programs and to make recommendations about implementing specific screening programs as well as to issue guidelines on existing ones. Their recommendations change over time, as new data on specific screening tests are disseminated. Inherent in this is a balance between the magnitude of the benefits of screening versus the magnitude of harms.

The U.S. Preventive Services Task Force, an independent, volunteer panel of national experts in disease prevention and evidence-based medicine, makes evidence-based recommendations about clinical preventive services, including screening for disease. The objective is not only to offer guidance to doctors and other health care providers but also to provide individuals with the most accurate and up-to-date information on ways to prevent illness and to improve health and well-being.[10] The Task Force assigns each recommendation a letter grade (an A, B, C, or D grade or an I-statement) based on the strength of the evidence and the balance of benefits and harms of a preventive service. An A grade means that the Task Force recommends screening because there is a high certainly that the net benefit will be substantial. A B grade means that the Task Force recommends the service because there is high certainty that the net benefit is moderate or that there is moderate certainty that the net benefit is moderate to substantial. A grade of C means that the net benefit is small, and a grade of D means that there is no net benefit to screening, or that the harms outweigh the benefits. A grade of I means that the current evidence is insufficient to assess the balance of benefits and harms of the service. The Task Force issues recommendations for a wide variety of clinical conditions, which are listed in Appendix A.

It would be incorrect, however, to assume that screening *per se* can protect a person from a disease. Getting screened will not prevent a disease from developing. The value of screening is to identify individuals who have abnormal test results that need to be further investigated and then, once the disease is confirmed clinically, proceed with appropriate treatment. This preventive measure could stop a disease from developing into something serious and perhaps even delay death.

Screening for cancer, the subject of this book, can be more problematic. Cancer is not one disease, and not every cancer should be screened for. In some cases, screening may actually do more harm than good by having the individual undergo many tests and procedures to rule in or rule out suspected cancer. In some instances, abnormal cells detected on screening would never progress to disease or death. Many men, for example, have malignant prostate cells at death. These malignant cells, although present, do not cause or contribute to death. They are indolent (e.g., slow growing) cells in which disease progresses slowly and does not pose an immediate or even long-term threat. The following chapter discusses cancer-specific screening, including the potential benefits and potential harms, in more depth.

Is Every Disease Appropriate for Screening?

Early detection of a disease is admirable but is not alone a sufficient reason to initiate a screening program. Why? Because not every disease would be appropriate for screening—for many different and important reasons. Which diseases should be screened? Which should not be screened? Some screening tests are considered to have a benefit, but in other cases, the benefits are less clear. How "good" is the test at detecting abnormal findings? Should everyone get screened or should the screening program only target those considered to be at higher risk for developing the disease? Screening should also demonstrate that people would live longer as a result of earlier detection and subsequent treatment. That is, will people who get screened have better survival rates than those who don't get screened? Other important questions need to be addressed, such as: How frequently should people be screened for a specific disease? Do the potential benefits outweigh the potential harms of screening? Further, there are economic, ethical, and clinical issues that must be considered before a screening program is implemented. Screening programs are usually costly exercises and do not always deliver the expected benefits in terms of improved health outcomes or longer life expectancy. In some instances, they can do more harm than good.

What Constitutes a "Good Screening Test"?

An ideal screening test should be considered for diseases and conditions that are considered "serious" if left untreated and are prevalent in the population (e.g., cervical, breast, and colon cancer; hypertension; diabetes; high cholesterol). There is very little point in screening for a disease that few people have (e.g., screening for gallstones). The screening test must identify a disease that is clinically significant and that, if left untreated, will cause significant morbidity and mortality. Further, the disease must have a preclinical phase, a presymptomatic stage, in which the disease is detectable. And, most importantly, there must be an acceptable treatment course for those who test positive and have the disease. The test should be reasonably priced, cost-effective, and preferably be noninvasive. Screening is very inefficient when the prevalence of the condition is low. One would not screen for HIV AIDS in the general population, for example. However, screening for this disease in a cohort deemed to be at high risk for this disease would make sense.

The purpose of screening, however, is not only to detect a condition but also to enable people to live longer (e.g., increase survival). Early detection by itself is probably insufficient to justify a screening program. There has to be evidence that screening contributes to survival, and this implies that there are treatments for the disease that would be available to those who test positive. If the treatment works just as well later in the course of the disease, screening for early detection probably is not warranted. The World Health Organization has gone on record in defining the criteria for population-based screening and makes the point that if early diagnosis and treatment does not lead to an improved health outcome, detecting disease earlier would make people worry and probably receive treatment unnecessarily because they would not benefit from early treatment.

Guidelines recommending screening are best if based on randomized clinical trials in which results from a screening program are compared to conventional care or to some gold standard. However, based on evidence from observational studies that show large benefits with a minimal downside, there really isn't a need for a clinical trial. Above all else, before a screening program is implemented, there must be a consensus based on the "best evidence" that the screening program will do more good than harm.

In summary, building on the Wilson and Jungner screening criteria, a "good" screening test should have the following characteristics:[11]

- The disease should be an important health problem. Screening should be done for diseases with serious consequences if left undetected and not treated. The screening test should potentially result in clear benefits to people's health.
- The disease should be sufficiently prevalent in the target population.
- The screening test should be sufficiently accurate to detect the disease at an early stage.
- There must be a treatment for the disease. It is unethical to initiate a screening program if the treatment required in order to act upon the results is not available.
- Early detection should lead to improved survival.
- Facilities for diagnosis and treatment must be available.
- The screening test should be acceptable to the target population.
- The screening test should be cost-effective.
- The screening test should be sufficiently sensitive and specific.
- The ethical imperative with all medical interventions is to ensure as far as possible that the potential benefits will outweigh the potential harms.

How "Good" Is a Screening Test?

A "good" screening test should accurately differentiate who has the disease and who does not. That is, the test should be sufficiently sensitive and sufficiently specific. Sensitivity is the ability of a test to correctly identify those with the disease (true positive rate), whereas specificity is the ability of the test to correctly identify those without the disease (true negative rate).

A test with 100% sensitivity correctly identifies all patients with the disease. A test with 80% sensitivity detects 80% of patients with the disease (true positives), but 20% with the disease will go undetected (false negatives). A sensitive test helps rule out disease when the result is negative. Conversely, a test with 100% specificity correctly identifies all patients without the disease. A test with 80% specificity correctly reports 80% of patients without the disease as test negative (true negatives), but 20% of the patients without the disease are incorrectly identified as test positive (false positives).

A test with high sensitivity is more likely to pick up most of those who actually have the disease, which is an important criterion for a screening test. A test with high specificity is unlikely to mislabel people as having the disease if they actually do not. A highly specific test means that there are few false positive results. There always is a trade-off between high sensitivity and high specificity. One looks for a balance between the two, which is why determining the cutoff point of a test is so important. Cutoff values are the dividing points on measuring scales where the test results are divided. Those results above the cutoff point would refer to those who test positive (e.g., abnormal) and results below the cutoff point to those who test negative (e.g., normal). An objective in deciding on a cutoff point is to strike the proper balance between false positives and false negatives.

In a perfect world, a "perfect test" is never positive in a patient who is disease free and is never negative in a patient who is in fact diseased. In the real world, this is rare. Thus, it is important to understand the rationale of selecting the cutoff point, which will differentiate test positivity from negativity. There are trade-offs in making this decision. In general, the higher the sensitivity, the lower the specificity, and vice versa.

There are two other important characteristics of a screening test: the positive predictive value (PPV) and the negative predictive value (NPV). Positive predictive value is the probability that subjects with a positive screening test truly have the disease. Negative predictive value is the probability that subjects with a negative screening test truly do not have the disease. Unlike sensitivity or specificity, PPV and NPV are influenced by the prevalence of disease in the population that is being tested. That is, a screening test is conducted in a population where the disease prevalence is high; it is more likely that persons who test positive truly have disease than if the test is performed in a population with low prevalence.

There are instances when a screening test should not be implemented. It could be that there is not a test that is sufficiently sensitive or specific to warrant screening. Or there are instances in which the disease would be detected at a late stage even with screening, thus obviating the benefits of screening (e.g., lung cancer). It could be that the disease is not amenable for screening because there aren't accurate screening tests that have been developed (e.g., ovarian cancer). It could be that the test is too expensive, or, for whatever reason, the general public views the test as being not acceptable (e.g., too invasive). In short, there are many reasons why screening for a specific disease would not be appropriate.

Types of Screening Programs

Screening programs come in many different forms. *Organized population-based screening programs* target a community/population in a geographic area, for example, a program to screen a population for hypertension or diabetes or glaucoma. The screening is available to all regardless of risk status. In contrast, high-risk screening programs target only those who are considered to be at higher risk for the disease. In a screening program for sickle cell anemia, for example, one would not screen the entire population because the disease is not prevalent among the general population. However, in specific population groups where the disease is known to be highly prevalent (i.e., African Americans), those at high risk for the disease should be screened.

Multiphasic community-based screening programs refer to the application of two or more screenings at one time instead of conducting separate screening tests for a single disease, for example, screening for common diseases such as hearing loss, hypertension, and diabetes at a "health fair." School-based screening programs are excellent means to screen school children for diseases and conditions such as hearing loss, vision, and dental problems.

Screening can also be used to protect a population from exposure to infectious disease (e.g., TB or HIV). The primary aim of this type of screening is not to benefit the individual per se, but to protect the local population. Those who test positive, for example, would be referred to a clinician for definitive diagnosis and then prescribed medication to hopefully prevent the spread of the disease in the general population. This type of screening relies on "case finding."

Another type of screening, *opportunistic screening*, is neither a formal nor an organized screening program. Rather, this type of screening is initiated by the individual or his/her health care provider during the physical exam. A population-based screening program is an organized, coordinated means of testing for disease in a large number of people.

Population-based screening is also different from *diagnostic screening*. The purpose of a diagnostic test is to establish the presence (or absence) of disease as a basis for treatment decisions in symptomatic or screen positive individuals. Unlike population-based screening tests, diagnostic tests are confirmatory tests. People go to the doctor because of symptoms, and diagnostic tests are run to determine what is causing the problem. Population-based screening tests are usually done on large numbers of asymptomatic, but potentially at-risk individuals, whereas diagnostic tests are done on symptomatic individuals to establish diagnosis or asymptomatic individuals with a positive screening test. These tests may be invasive and expensive.

Genetic screening is the newest form of screening, made possible by advances in technology. The purpose of genetic screening is to identify individuals who are at risk for a genetic disease or for transmitting a gene for a genetic disease. For example, prenatal genetic testing refers to tests that are done during pregnancy to either screen for or diagnose a birth defect. Screening tests, such as amniocentesis and alpha fetoprotein testing, can determine whether the baby is more or less likely to have certain birth defects or genetic disorders (e.g., Down syndrome). Based on this information, expectant parents and their medical team make informed decisions and choices.

Genetic screening is done on an individual, not population-based, level and, as such, is different from the other types of screening just described. Since the 1990s, genetic screening has been used to identify mutations in genes that could lead to various cancers. One form of breast cancer that is strongly hereditary can be identified by mutations in genes (*BRCA1* and *BRCA2*), which significantly increases the risk of breast cancer among those who have this mutation. Similar predisposing genes were later found for a form of colorectal cancer as well as certain types of cardiovascular disease.

Genetic test results are not always straightforward, which can make them challenging to interpret and explain. A positive test result may confirm a diagnosis, indicating that a person is a carrier of a particular genetic mutation, identify an increased risk of developing a disease in the future, or may even suggest a need for further testing. Positive test results do not establish the exact risk of developing a disorder. Also, health professionals typically cannot use a positive test result to predict the course or severity of a condition. On the other hand, a negative test result may mean that the laboratory did not find a change in the gene, chromosome, or protein under consideration. This result could indicate that a person is not affected by a particular disorder, is not a carrier of a specific genetic mutation, or does not have an increased risk of developing a certain disease. However, it is possible that the test missed a disease-causing genetic alteration; many genetic tests cannot detect all genetic changes that can cause a particular disorder, which implies that further testing may be required to confirm a negative result.

There is ongoing, exciting research in gene therapy and precision or personalized medicine as well as pharmacological research on drugs targeted specifically at mutation carriers. However, so far, the benefits of genetic testing in preventing or managing particular diseases have been mixed.[12] This topic will be discussed in more detail in a subsequent chapter.

It is important to understand that genetic testing often cannot determine if a person will show symptoms of a disorder, provide an indication of how severe the symptoms will be should they present, or to what extent the disease or disorder will progress over time. Another major limitation is the lack of treatment strategies for many genetic disorders once they are diagnosed (e.g., Huntington's disease, Alzheimer's disease). And the issue of genetic discrimination should an employer or an insurance company find out about the test results may put some people off from being tested for inherited diseases even though in 2008 Congress passed the Genetic Information Nondiscrimination Act.

Regardless of the type of screening program, the objectives are the same: to identify individuals who are at high risk of developing a disease and should be referred for further testing in order to make a definitive diagnosis and to initiate appropriate treatment. Recommendations for specific screening tests will vary by age, gender, race/ethnicity, and disease risk factors. As stated earlier, not everyone would be a good candidate for a specific screening program. Individuals targeted for screening should be those in whom the prevalence of the disease, or the risk of developing the disease, is substantial enough to warrant screening. One would not screen for sexually transmitted diseases in a population that is not sexually active, for example.

Limitations of Screening

There are several pitfalls in screening that must be taken into account. In particular, two types of errors can and do occur: the test result may incorrectly show a positive result when in fact the individual does not have the disease (false positive). Conversely, the test may be negative when in fact the individual does have the disease (false negative). Other limitations of screening programs can include: stress and anxiety caused by the false positive screening test result; unnecessary investigation and treatment of false positive results; cost of further diagnostic testing/workup; and a false sense of security caused by false negatives, which may end up delaying diagnosis and treatment. Weighing the potential benefits of the screening program against the potential harms is imperative.

Screening also may lead to overdiagnosis and overtreatment for individuals in whom the disease would not have posed a problem had the screening test not identified the "problem." Overdiagnosis refers to disease that will almost never cause symptoms or death during a patient's lifetime. These are referred to as "harmless abnormalities." That is, some cancers are slow growing and best left alone, but if a screening test is positive, there is an ethical mandate to order tests to diagnose the problem definitively, which often leads to unnecessary, costly treatment.

The effectiveness of early treatment is among one of the more important factors to consider when deciding whether to screen or not. If effective treatment is not available, ethically one should not screen for the disease in the first place. For a screening program to be beneficial (e.g., improve health outcomes, increase life expectancy), it must include a treatment that is not only effective but also is more effective if applied earlier rather than later. If the treatment works just as well later in the course of the disease, screening for early detection is not necessary.

Lead time and *length time bias* are two issues that also need to be taken into account when assessing the impact of a screening program. Lead time bias refers to the length of time between the detection of a disease and its clinical presentation and diagnosis. It is the time between early diagnosis with screening and the time in which diagnosis would have been made without screening. That is, the disease is detected earlier in its natural history with screening. Survival appears to be increased because the disease is detected earlier in the natural history. The survival time since diagnosis is longer with screening, but life span is not been prolonged. Screening appears to increase survival time (lead time), but those with the disease, whether they were screened or not, die at the same time. As such, lead time bias may distort screening's ability to save lives.

Length time bias is often discussed in the context of the benefits of cancer screening. Length time bias refers to the situation when slow-growing, less aggressive disease is detected by screening. These cancers remain in the body longer than fast-growing cancers before symptoms develop, which can lead to the perception that screening leads to better outcomes when in reality it has no effect. For example, some breast cancers detected in a screening program may be less aggressive, slower-growing than those diagnosed when symptoms appear. The length of time that a cancer is detectable by screening is greater for the slow-growing tumors. That is, slower-growing tumors have better prognoses than tumors with faster-growing tumors.

In this example, screening is more likely to detect slower-growing tumors, which may be less deadly than faster-growing tumors. Thus, screening may tend to detect cancers that would not have killed the patient or even been detected prior to death from other causes. The malignant cells probably would have caused no harm or required treatment over the course of the individual's lifetime.

For example, a patient may survive for 10 years after clinical diagnosis at age 50 or survive for 15 years after the screening-detected diagnosis at age 45. However, this simply reflects earlier diagnosis, because the overall survival time of the patient is unchanged, and there is actually no benefit from screening in terms of survival. The person still died at age 60 but knew about the disease for five years before it was clinically detected. In this example of survival from diagnosis, there is a lead time bias of five years, which constitutes an artificial addition to the survival time of screen-detected cases.

Length time bias is different in that it refers to situations with more slowly growing tumors that are less likely to be fatal. They may have a longer presymptomatic, screen-detectable period, which means that the disease would be more likely to be screen-detected, and this could confer an artificial survival advantage. For example, if the same number of slow-growing and fast-growing tumors appear in a year, the screening test will detect the more slow-growing tumors rather than the faster-growing ones. If the slow-growing tumors are less likely to be fatal than the fast growers, the people whose cancer is detected by screening do better, on average, than the people whose tumors are detected from symptoms (or at autopsy) even if there is no real benefit to early diagnosis. Screening appears to lead to better survival even if no effective treatment is given. Length time bias is due to slow cases being detected more often simply because they are slowly progressing.

Balancing the Potential Benefits against the Potential Harms of Screening

It is important to understand the advantages and disadvantages of screening, as well as the balance of benefits and harmful effects from the screening test. Some screening tests are more benign than others. For example, screening for glaucoma or high blood pressure is done by simple-to-administer, inexpensive, low-risk tests with potentially high value. Screening for colon cancer, for example, is an invasive and expensive test although it is probably the "best" test to screen for this type of cancer.

When deciding on whether to get screened for a disease, it is important to know if you are at higher risk of getting the disease because of age, ethnicity/race, genetics, and lifestyle. The higher the risk, the more important it is to be screened. When deciding whether to be screened, there are some questions that one should consider. For example, is the test appropriate for me at my age/race/ethnicity? How likely is it that I could develop the disease? To what extent would I benefit from screening in the long term (e.g., what do studies show about survival rates among those screened compared to those not screened)? If I test positive on the screening test, are there treatments available? How sensitive and specific is the screening test? How common are false positive test results? How common are false negative test results? How expensive is the test? How often will I have to have a screening test in order to benefit from screening?

Screening for cancer is not necessarily straightforward. As evidence accumulates, we are getting a better understanding that more screening does not necessarily translate into fewer cancer deaths and that some screening may actually do more harm than good. The following chapters discuss several cancer screening modalities, paying particular attention to the potential benefits versus the potential harms.

CHAPTER FOUR

Screening for Cancer: The Pros and Cons

Most people know someone who has had cancer and maybe even died of the disease. Cancer is the most common human genetic disease and in many respects is unlike other diseases for which screening tests are recommended primarily because cancer embodies a host of medical, surgical, and psychological issues that are different from other diseases. Individuals who have cancer experience a variety of physical and psychological illness-related factors that affect quality of life (for them and their loved ones) in unique ways. The diagnosis of cancer evokes fear in many people. Many individuals find the thought of "cancer" to be scary.

Most cancers last a long time, requiring intense treatment often with serious side effects, including physical, physiological, and psychological. Unlike other diseases, those undergoing cancer treatment are often described as "coping with cancer" or "living with cancer". Those who successfully complete cancer treatment are often referred to as "cancer survivors." Yet, some "cancer survivors" may go into remission only to have the cancer return.

Lung, breast, colorectal, prostate, and stomach cancers are the top five leading types of cancer globally. Lung cancer is the most common cancer in men worldwide followed by prostate, colorectal, and stomach cancer. Breast cancer is the most common cancer in women worldwide followed by colorectal, lung, and cervical cancer.[1]

The following shows the number of new cases diagnosed in 2018 and the percentage of all cancers (excluding nonmelanoma skin cancer) for the top five cancers worldwide.

1. Lung: new cases—2,093,876 (12.3% of all cancers)
2. Breast: new cases—2,088,849 (12.3% of all cancers)
3. Colorectal: new cases—1,800,977 (10.6% of all cancers)
4. Prostate: new cases—1,276,106 (7.5% of all cancers)
5. Stomach: new cases—1,033,701 (6.1% of all cancers)

Cancer is a leading cause of death worldwide, accounting for an estimated 9.6 million deaths in 2018. Globally, the World Health Organization (WHO) estimates that 1 in 6 deaths is due to cancer.[2] Tobacco use is the most important risk factor for cancer and is responsible for approximately 22% of cancer deaths. Cancer-causing infections such as hepatitis B and C and human papilloma virus (HPV) are responsible for approximately 25% of cancer cases in low- and middle-income countries (LMICs), where late-stage presentation, diagnosis, and treatment are common.[3]

Some cancers, if diagnosed at an early stage, are more likely to respond to treatment, which can result in a greater probability of survival. The primary goal is to diagnose the cancer and initiate treatment that hopefully will lead to a cure for the cancer or to considerably prolong life.

It is a commonly held belief among health professionals that early detection of cancer is beneficial; ergo, screening for cancer is a good thing to do. If a malignancy is found early, it may be easier to treat or cure. Conversely, by the time symptoms appear, the cancer may have grown and spread, making it much more difficult to treat. The thinking is that with detection of cancer at an early stage the prognosis for survival should be better than if there was no screening. Given that the cancer would be "caught early," the likelihood that an individual would not die from the disease, at least in the short term, is expected. But in some instances, cancer screening does not necessarily translate into fewer cancer deaths, and some screening tests may actually cause more harm than good, which is why it is important for people to be aware of the potential benefits of a particular cancer screening test as well as the potential harms. Questions that should be considered include: Is getting screened going to be beneficial to me? If the answer is yes, how so? What happens if the test is positive? Understanding the potential benefits and potential harms of cancer screening must take into consideration what would happen after a positive screening test result. As explained in the previous chapter, a test positive result requires diagnostic testing to rule in or rule out cancer.

Because most cancer screening tests themselves are generally noninvasive, harms from the test itself are typically minor. That is the good news. However, there are some cancer screening tests that are invasive and could lead to test-related complications (e.g., perforation with colonoscopy). Follow-up invasive diagnostic procedures, such as a biopsy, are also associated with low but possible risks of complications. These tests/procedures, many of which are invasive, can be costly, and waiting for the results may cause anxiety. Further, the workup could detect a cancer that would be best handled by doing nothing. The cancer may never become clinically apparent in the absence of screening, causing no harm to the individual. It may also turn out that there is no evidence of cancer (a false positive test result), which of course would be received as a welcome relief. But this news has to be confirmed by additional tests and procedures.

Screening for Cancer

Over the years, considerable debate and discussion of the value of cancer screening focused on which cancers to screen, on whom, at what age, and how frequently. Also, and importantly, to what extent does screening reduce mortality from the disease? Consider a woman in her early 40s with an average risk of breast cancer. Naturally she would want to have a cancer detected at an early stage. Should she have a mammogram in her early 40s? Should she wait until age 50 as recommended by several breast cancer screening guidelines? How frequently after the first mammogram should subsequent screening be scheduled thereafter? Annually? Every two years? To what extent does early breast cancer screening save lives? The answers to these questions are not straightforward, especially since there is ongoing debate regarding the appropriate age at which routine mammography screening should begin. Although the data do not provide a clear indication that screening women at younger ages (e.g., less than 50 years) is beneficial, clearly many factors (e.g., genetics, demographics, the biology of the disease, and patient preference) need to be taken into account in the decision-making. Subsequent chapters will discuss breast cancer screening in more depth.

Other cancer screening tests also have led to controversy and uncertainty. The debate over when men of a certain age should have a prostate-specific antigen (PSA) screening test, for example, has created confusion within the medical profession as well as the public. How accurate is this test? Are there "too many" false positive tests that make the PSA test an unreliable means of screening for prostate cancer? At what age should a man have a PSA test? Should he have this test at all? What happens if the PSA level is elevated? Should the test be repeated after a period of time to see if the PSA level is still high?

As with breast cancer screening, many factors must be taken into account in deciding who would benefit the most from PSA screening and who might not. Prostate cancer is a slow-growing, localized cancer. An elevated PSA reading usually triggers diagnostic testing to determine the next best course of action, which could lead to overdiagnosis and overtreatment, issues that have clouded the value of this particular screening test. In some cases, the

PSA test detects abnormal cells that would never have progressed to cause symptoms or complications or even death. The potential harms of screening need to be balanced against the potential benefits. Would foregoing the PSA test be a better course of action for some men?

Not all cancers would be appropriate for screening. While there are sensitive and specific screening tests for several cancers, for others such tests do not exist at this time. That is, there may not be a sufficiently sensitive and specific screening test available to detect the cancer at an early stage. For example, stomach cancer globally is a leading cause of death, but a good screening test does not exist at this time. A screening test to detect early-stage ovarian cancer, a leading cause of death among women, is also lacking. There are, however, several types of cancer for which the benefits of screening outweigh the potential risks or harms of not detecting the cancer at an early stage. Screening tests for cervical and oral cancer, for example, are easy to administer, are not particularly invasive, and are inexpensive. But most importantly, these cancers, if detected at an early stage, have an excellent prognosis in terms of survival. The same can be said for screening for colorectal cancer, although the "gold standard" test, colonoscopy, is invasive and costly.

Cervical Cancer Screening

Cervical cancer, a relatively slow-growing cancer, is the fourth leading cause of death among women worldwide, but is the leading cause of cancer mortality among women living in LMICs. There were an estimated 570,000 new cases in 2018, representing 6.6% of all female cancers. However, approximately 90% of deaths from cervical cancer occurred in LMICs.[4] These women—mothers, wives, grandmothers—are in their most productive years of life and contribute economically to the family welfare. Death from cervical cancer leaves a large gap in the fabric of the family. The numbers clearly show that women in LMICs are disproportionately represented in cervical cancer mortality statistics.

The striking global health inequity, resulting in higher morbidity and mortality of women living in LMICs (especially sub-Saharan Africa and Southeastern Asia) compared to women living in high-income countries (e.g., the developed world), can be overcome if all women between the ages of 30 and 65 get screened. (Note: screening recommendations will vary among developed countries and LMICs.) The primary reason for this disparity is that women in high-income countries are routinely screened for cervical cancer, whereas those in the LMICs are not. The sad thing is that cervical cancer is both preventable and curable if diagnosed in its early stage. Survival rates for cervical cancer, especially for cancer detected in the early stage, correlate highly with early detection and treatment.

There are several known risk factors for cervical cancer, including having many sexual partners; beginning sexual activity at an early age; having sexually transmitted infections (STIs)—such as chlamydia, gonorrhea, syphilis, and HIV/AIDS; and tobacco smoking. These are factors that could elevate the risk of developing cervical cancer, but do not guarantee *per se* that an individual will develop cancer. That being said, nearly all cases of cervical cancer can be attributed to HPV infection, including HPV types 16 and 18, which cause most cases of cervical cancer. HPV infection is the strongest predictor of cervical cancer; however, having a HPV infection does not mean that a woman will automatically develop cervical cancer. Rather, she is at higher risk because of the infection. The strong association between cervical cancer and HPV makes testing for HPV a valuable and important cervical cancer screening tool.

In the developed world, screening for cervical cancer relies on the Pap test (also called Pap smear), where cells are collected from the cervix and tested in a cytology lab. The Pap test detects abnormal cervical cells, including precancerous cervical lesions, as well as early cervical cancers. The American Cancer Society Cervical Cancer Screening Guidelines recommend that women in the United States between the ages of 21 and 29 should have a Pap test every three years. Women between the ages of 30 and 65 should have both a Pap test and an HPV test every five years or a Pap test alone every three years. Women over age 65 who have had regular screening tests with normal results no longer need to be screened; however, women who are considered to be at high risk might benefit from continued screening.[5]

Because many LMICs lack high-quality cytology labs and trained technicians to read the slides, the Pap test is often not feasible, especially in rural areas. Also, the cost of the test is usually too high for most rural and urban women in LMICs to afford. Fortunately, a low-tech option has been shown to be highly effective in detecting abnormal cervical cells. Visual inspection with acetic acid (VIA) has been shown repeatedly to be an excellent, inexpensive alternative to cytology-based screening. The test relies on vinegar (i.e., acetic acid) and does not have to be performed by a physician! Abnormal cells in the cervix will turn white within approximately 10 seconds after application of the vinegar solution. Women who test positive can receive treatment at the time of visit (e.g., cryotherapy). Based on evidence from many low-tech cervical cancer screening programs in LMICs, the WHO concluded that VIA is a simple, safe, feasible, and effective screening test and should be used in LMICs.[6] Despite the availability of VIA in LMICs, screening remains uneven and low, especially in rural areas. Reasons for this include economics, lack of knowledge about cervical cancer and the benefits of screening, accessibility and availability of testing sites, and trained health personnel.

In 2013, the WHO recommended that LMICs use a strategy of screening with an HPV test followed by VIA.[7] In areas where the Pap test is used, the WHO recommended that the preferred way to find early cervical cancers or precancers in women aged 30 and older is by Pap test plus an HPV test (called co-testing). For women aged 30 and older, both HPV/Pap co-testing and HPV testing alone are more sensitive than Pap testing alone. Therefore, a woman with a negative HPV test and normal Pap test—or just a negative HPV test—has a very low risk of developing precancerous cervical lesions over the next several years.[8]

Advances in molecular genetics are providing a better understanding of the natural history of HPV infection at the molecular level.[9] Molecular HPV testing is being developed as the next generation of cervical cancer screening and is showing great promise. For example, a well-designed study showed that screening women with a single round of HPV DNA testing was associated with a significant reduction in the numbers of advanced cervical cancers and deaths from this cancer.[10] Evidence shows that a single negative HPV DNA test provides five to ten years of confidence against a high-grade precancerous cervical lesion.[11] Technology has advanced to the point that women can test themselves by means of self-collection of HPV test samples. A woman can collect vaginal samples in the comfort and privacy of her home. Self-testing is a potentially promising strategy for reaching women who have not been routinely screened for cervical cancer and could help overcome cultural barriers to going to a clinic or doctor's office for a gynecologic exam.

In terms of preventing cervical cancer, an HPV vaccine is considered to be the single most effective way to prevent cervical cancer. Several HPV vaccines have been brought to market since 2006. These vaccines can prevent infection from the types of HPV most likely to cause cancer and genital warts and are most effective when given to children (preteen and teen), preferably before they become sexually active. A 2019 large-scale global study that includes data from 60 million individuals and up to eight years of postvaccination follow-up found compelling evidence of the substantial impact of HPV vaccination programs on HPV infections and cervical cancer (e.g., CIN2+) among girls and women.[12] The results provide strong evidence of HPV vaccination's impact; specifically, the two types of HPV that cause 70% of cervical cancers (HPV 16 and 18) were significantly reduced after vaccination. However, the lack of data from LMICs, where the burden of disease is far greater than in high-income countries, makes it difficult to assess the benefits of the vaccine in these countries, and the researchers state that the results should be extrapolated to those countries with caution.

Unfortunately at this point in time in many LMICs, and even in the United States, the cost of the HPV vaccination is such that many are unable to afford the vaccination. Given the findings from the 2019 study, however, efforts should be made to enable young girls to be vaccinated. The potential benefits far outweigh any reasons why vaccination should not be provided. From a global policy perspective, the results of this study serve to reinforce the WHO's recommendation that HPV vaccination be implemented widely in an effort to eliminate cervical cancer, especially in LMICs.

Although guidelines differ on when a woman should be screened, how frequently, and whether she lives in a developed country or an LMIC, the evidence is solid that cervical cancer screening saves lives. However, as with any screening program, it is imperative that there is a referral process in place for women who test positive. Further there should be a mechanism in place to provide treatment, including cryotherapy, colposcopy, or loop electrosurgical excision procedure (LEEP) for those who test positive. Those who need more extensive procedures (e.g., hysterectomy) should be referred to a tertiary hospital for care.

In 2018, the WHO made a global call for action to eliminate cervical cancer.[13] The evidence from numerous studies shows that most of the cases of cervical cancer deaths could have been prevented had women been screened and the disease detected at an early stage. Given what we know about cervical cancer prevention and treatment, no woman should have to die from this disease.

Oral Cancer Screening

While cancers of the breast, cervix, colon, and prostate are the focus of most cancer prevention screening programs, the relatively high incidence of oral cavity cancer, particularly in LMICs, highlights the need for screening for this cancer. Oral cancer comprises a subset of head and neck cancers, which can appear in any part of the mouth. The overwhelming majority of cases arise from the epithelial lining as squamous cell carcinomas.

Oral cancer, the 11th most common cancer in the world, is more prevalent in males and is much more common in LMICs. There are approximately 650,000 new cases and 330,000 deaths annually, but this is probably an underestimate because of underreporting in many LMICs.[14] Unfortunately, oral cancer is usually fatal primarily because most cases are diagnosed in the advanced stages despite the fact that it is a preventable form of cancer and easily treatable when diagnosed in the early stages.

There is a wide geographical variation (approximately 20-fold) in the reporting of oral cancer incidence of this cancer with South and Southeast Asia (e.g., Sri Lanka, India, Pakistan, and Taiwan), Western (e.g., France) and Eastern Europe (e.g., Hungary, Slovakia, and Slovenia), some countries in Latin America and the Caribbean (e.g., Brazil, Uruguay, and Puerto Rico), and the Pacific region (e.g., Papua New Guinea and Melanesia) having the highest rates.[15] The primary treatment for this cancer is surgery followed by radiation and/or chemotherapy.

Major risk factors for oral cancer include smoking tobacco products (cigarettes, cigars, pipes) and nonsmoking products (chewing tobacco); betel nut chewing, which is widespread in certain regions of Asia; alcohol consumption; HPV; and the herpes simplex virus (HSV). HPV has been identified in almost one-quarter of all oral cancer cases.

Screening for oral cancer is easy, cheap, and noninvasive. A dentist, doctor, or trained nurse looks for swellings, bumps, unusual patches of color, ulcerations, or other abnormalities in the oral cavity. The point is that screening for oral cancer should be routinely done so as to identify abnormalities at an early, treatable stage. Early diagnosis and treatment of oral cancer could positively influence survival.

Colorectal Cancer Screening

Colorectal cancer is a slowly developing malignancy, the vast majority (over 95%) of which are classified as adenocarcinomas. Colorectal cancer almost always develops from precancerous polyps (abnormal growths) in the colon or rectum. Most polyps, common in people older than 50 years of age, are not cancerous; however, a certain type of polyp (adenoma) may have a higher risk of becoming a cancer. Removing these substantially reduces the risk of colorectal cancer developing.

Colorectal cancer is the third most common cancer in men, and the fourth in women, with 1.8 million new cases and almost 861,000 deaths in 2018.[16] Australia and New Zealand, Europe, and North America have the highest rates of this cancer, and African and South-Central Asian countries have the lowest. Colorectal cancer is uncommon before the age of 40, but increases significantly between the ages of 40 and 50. Only recently has the incidence of colorectal cancer in men and women under the age of 50 in the United States been steadily increasing (at a rate of 2% per year from 1992 through 2013), although the number of new cases in this age group remains far lower than for adults aged 50 and over. The reasons for this are not clear.[17] Moreover, there are differences among racial/ethnic groups, with African Americans having the highest rate of colorectal cancer.

Overall death rates from colorectal cancer have declined since the mid-1980s in the United States and in many other Western countries, which can be explained in part by early detection and removal of precancerous polyps.[18] The United States has one of the highest survival rates from colorectal cancer; however, mortality rates continue to increase in other countries (e.g., Central and South America and Eastern Europe).

There are several factors that increase the risk of developing colorectal cancer, including genetics and family history, obesity, cigarette smoking, excessive alcohol consumption, and a red meat/high-fat diet. Further, individuals with inflammatory bowel disease, including chronic ulcerative colitis and Crohn's disease, are at higher risk compared to those who do not have these conditions. There are also several factors that have been shown to be somewhat associated with a decreased risk of colorectal cancer, including regular physical activity, eating a high fiber diet and a diet rich in vegetables (especially cruciferous vegetables such as broccoli and cauliflower), and the regular use of aspirin or nonsteroidal anti-inflammatory drugs (NSAIDs).[19] However, the strength of association of these potential risk factors with the development of colorectal cancer is not as strong as that for the other more proven risk factors.

Screening for colorectal cancer involves testing for precancerous colorectal polyps or early-stage cancer before symptoms appear, before the disease has a chance to grow or spread. Treatment is easier to manage, less expensive, and more likely to be successful at an early stage. Because the vast majority of new cases of colorectal cancer (about 90%) occur in people who are 50 and older, screening is more appropriate in this age cohort than in younger age cohorts. Although various guidelines differ slightly regarding the recommended age of first screening, all recommend that people should be screened for colorectal cancer.

The American Cancer Society colorectal cancer screening guidelines recommend that adults at average risk should begin regular colorectal screening at age 45, but those with a family history or other risk factors should talk with their doctor about beginning earlier.[20] The U.S. Preventive Services Task Force recommends that men and women between the ages of 50 and 75 be screened for colorectal cancer.[21] Recommendations generally advocate having a colonoscopy every 10 years for those at low risk for the disease. Individuals who have a higher risk for developing colorectal cancer should be screened earlier, and those at higher risk should be screened more frequently rather than waiting 10 years between screenings.

There are several good screening tests for colorectal cancer. The flexible fiberoptic sigmoidoscope, introduced in 1969 as a screening tool for an examination of the distal colon, was an improvement over the rigid sigmoidoscope, which is not able to detect as many polyps as the flexible scope. Having a sigmoidoscopy requires pretest preparation, but there is no need for sedation. Today, colonoscopy is the mainstay of colon cancer screening. Unlike sigmoidoscopy in which only the rectum and sigmoid colon are examined, colonoscopy permits viewing of the entire colon. During this procedure, the doctor is able to take a biopsy and remove any polyps. Colonoscopies require a thorough cleansing of the colon before the test, and individuals are lightly sedated during the procedure. Unlike sigmoidoscopy, colonoscopy is expensive, but most U.S. health insurance plans will cover some of the costs of the procedure.

Virtual colonoscopy, also called computerized tomography (CT) colonography, is a newer way to screen for polyps. This procedure uses x-rays and a computer to create images of the rectum and colon from outside the body without the need for sedation. Virtual colonoscopy can show the presence of ulcers, polyps, and cancer. Pretest preparation, however, is necessary for this test. While there are fewer risks of virtual colonoscopy compared to regular colonoscopy, if polyps or other abnormal growths are seen, the individual will have to undergo a colonoscopy. The extent to which virtual colonoscopy should be used as a screening tool will depend on an individual's risk factors for the disease. But the combination of virtual colonoscopy screening with regular colonoscopy follow-up could be a cost-effective effort to increase colorectal cancer screening, especially in low-risk individuals.

There are other less expensive (and less invasive) tests available to screen for colorectal cancer, including the Fecal Occult Blood Test (FOBT), which can detect blood in the stool using a guaiac-based assay and is relatively inexpensive, convenient, and easy to administer. Polyps in the colon and small cancers can cause small amounts of bleeding, which could be an indication of cancer. The next generation of tests uses immunochemical-based testing. The fecal immunochemical test (iFOBT and FIT) uses antibodies to detect blood in the stool, and the FIT-DNA test (e.g., Cologuard®) combines the FIT test with a test that detects altered DNA in the stool. While these tests can identify abnormalities that could be cancerous, the removal of polyps, for example, is not possible. One would need to have a colonoscopy to do that.

The benefits of screening are only realized if people agree to be screened. Given the invasive nature of the colonoscopy and its costs, individuals may object to this form of screening. Hence, for those not considered to be at risk for this cancer, getting screened initially by one of the less invasive tests would be beneficial. Those at higher risk should have a colonoscopy, but those at lesser risk might be just as well off by having an FBOT or an FIT screen. The objective is to encourage as many people as possible to get screened because there is solid evidence that screening for colorectal cancer reduces colorectal mortality by approximately 60 to 70%.[22]

Prostate Cancer Screening

Prostate cancer, a slow-growing malignancy, can often be effectively treated and managed if detected by screening in its early stage. Prostate cancer is the most common malignancy among males worldwide. It is estimated that a man's lifetime risk of developing prostate cancer is 1 in 7.[23] It is not an uncommon or rare cancer, as each year 1.6 million men are diagnosed with and 366,000 men die of prostate cancer.[24] There is substantial geographic variation in the incidence, with prostate cancer much more prevalent in the developed world compared to LMICs, perhaps because of the lack of screening and/or the paucity of valid data showing the incidence and prevalence in

LMICs. It could be that there is a larger proportion of slow-growing cancers diagnosed in countries with PSA screening and, conversely, later presentation of disease in countries with limited screening.[25]

Prostate mortality rates are higher in LMICs, with the highest prostate cancer mortality rates among populations in the Caribbean and in Middle and Southern Africa. In contrast, the lowest prostate cancer mortality rates are observed in Asia, particularly in Eastern and South-Central Asia. That being said, trends in mortality are a function of changes in the incidence of prostate cancer as well as survival among patients. Although there is a high incidence of prostate cancer, there also is a long survival period. This means that men are being diagnosed with prostate cancer but are surviving/living longer with the disease.[26]

Studies have identified several major risk factors, including age, race/ethnicity, positive family history of prostate cancer, and a Western diet (e.g., high in saturated fats, red meats, and dairy products). It is rare for men younger than 40 years of age to develop prostate cancer, but one's risk dramatically increases after age 55. Regarding race/ethnicity, there is a threefold difference in incidence rates of prostate cancer across race/ethnicity groups in the United States, with the highest incidence observed among African American men. Further, men with a father or brother diagnosed with prostate cancer are at a two- to three-fold higher risk of being diagnosed, and the risk is nearly nine-fold higher for men with both.[27] Other factors may also increase the risk of developing prostate cancer risk, including obesity, physical activity, sexual activity, smoking, and occupation, but the association of these risk factors and development of cancer is weaker than the other risk factors mentioned. Conversely, several studies suggest that the consumption of vegetables and fruit is associated with a lower risk (e.g., protective effect) of developing prostate cancer.[28]

The digital rectal exam (DRE) had been the traditional screening method for prostate cancer, but this was acknowledged to be a poor predictor of cancer. The introduction of PSA testing was a substantial improvement in prostate cancer detection; however, PSA correlates only with the *risk of cancer.*

Blood PSA levels were first used to screen for prostate cancer in 1987, and approval for PSA as a screening test by the Food and Drug Administration (FDA) followed seven years later. PSA levels are also used to evaluate the results of prostate cancer treatment, and PSA readings are also used to estimate the severity of benign prostatic hyperplasia (BPH), nonmalignant enlargement of the gland.

Advances in prostate screening, including the PSA test, have led to a shift in the diagnosis and management of this cancer. That being said, while many, if not most, men will develop a slow-growing or indolent form of this cancer by the time they reach their 60s and older, there will be others who are diagnosed with an aggressive form and have a worse prognosis.

The controversy surrounding the PSA test focuses on what is considered to be a normal value. The issue of what is a "normal level" of PSA and an "abnormal level" continues to be discussed and debated. PSA values tend to rise with age, even in healthy men, and each man might have his own normal. For example, there are factors that typically produce a substantial and/or sustained rise in the PSA, including BPH, prostatitis, urinary tract infections, and even prostate biopsies. Moreover, the PSA test cannot differentiate slow-growing, indolent, harmless prostate cancers from the less common, aggressive, potentially lethal cancers. A biopsy would have to be done to do so.

An elevated PSA level does not necessarily mean that cancer is present. Many men diagnosed with prostate cancer have a normal PSA level. Hence, concern has been voiced that the PSA test has led to overdetection and overtreatment given the questionable accuracy of the PSA test. That is, without the PSA screening test, it is conceivable that the cancer would neither have been diagnosed nor have caused death.

Medical experts are divided regarding the benefits of PSA screening in saving lives. Results from a large-scale study conducted over 10 years, however, found that doing a PSA test on men with no symptoms does not save lives.[29] Another study came to an opposite conclusion.[30] Hence, there is uncertainty and disagreement about PSA testing recommendation.

The U.S. Preventive Services Task Force reviewed evidence on the benefits and harms of PSA-based screening and treatment of screen-detected prostate cancer and concluded that PSA-based screening in men aged 55 to 69 years prevents approximately 1.3 deaths from prostate cancer over 13 years per 1,000 men screened and 3 cases of metastatic cancer per 1,000 men screened, with no reduction in all-cause mortality. No benefit was found for PSA-based screening in men aged 70 years and older.[31] On the basis of its review, the Task Force concluded that the decision for men aged 55 to 69 years to have PSA-based screening should be an individual one and should include a discussion of the potential benefits and harms.

The American Cancer Screening Guidelines recommend that men who are at average risk of prostate cancer should discuss the possible risks and benefits of prostate cancer screening with their doctor before deciding whether to be screened starting at age 50. For those at higher risk (e.g., African American men and men who have a father or brother diagnosed with prostate cancer), a discussion should take place at age 45.[32]

In a sense, the PSA-based screening test is a double-edged sword. PSA testing has led to early detection of prostate cancer; however, this has not necessarily translated into survival or mortality benefit and may actually cause harm in terms of overtreatment, which may lead to treatment-related side effects, psychological distress, and financial costs. Until a "better" test is developed, the PSA test, with all its flaws, is the "best" prostate cancer screening tool available.

Lung Cancer Screening

Usually symptoms of lung cancer do not appear until the disease is already at an advanced, noncurable stage. Even though lung cancer is the most common cancer worldwide, as of this writing, the only recommended screening test is low-dose computed tomography (low-dose CT [LDCT] scan), an expensive test that requires skilled personnel to administer. It would not be an appropriate test to use for population-based screening. As such, the U.S. Preventive Services Task Force recommends annual screening for those who have a history of heavy smoking (e.g., a smoking history of 30 pack years or more) and for those who smoke now or have quit within the past 15 years.[33] Smoking is the leading risk factor for lung cancer, hence the recommendation for lung cancer screening only for those at high risk of developing the disease because of their smoking history and age.

Does screening for lung cancer make a difference in survival? The National Lung Screening Trial (NLST) compared two ways of detecting lung cancer: low-dose helical computed tomography (LDCT) and standard chest x-ray in 53,454 current or former heavy smokers aged 55 to 74. Key findings showed that people who got low-dose CT scan had a 15 to 20% lower chance of dying from lung cancer compared to those who only had chest x-rays. However, some other trials have not found a benefit from lung cancer screening.[34] None of the studies included people who never smoked.

Given that there is not an inexpensive screening test for lung cancer, and given that the evidence about the long-term benefits of screening is debatable, the American Cancer Society recommends that people who are at high risk for developing the disease (e.g., long-term smokers) talk with their physician about whether to get screened.[35] Population-based lung cancer screening, which would include healthy, low-risk individuals, would not be advisable based on what we know about this disease and the ability to detect abnormalities in the lung at an early stage.

Does Cancer Screening Save Lives?

One of the major purposes of screening is to detect disease at an early, more treatable stage and to increase survival. The evidence clearly shows that screening for cervical, oral, and colorectal cancer does make a difference, but the evidence for prostate and lung cancer is less clear. The truly reliable way to know if a cancer screening test reduces deaths is through a randomized clinical trial that would show a reduction in cancer deaths in individuals assigned to screening compared to those assigned to a control group (e.g., no screening). In reality, such trials are not always conducted for ethical or economic reasons. Further, there is misunderstanding among physicians about 5-year survival (e.g., people who will be alive after five years after diagnosis).

One survey found that most primary care physicians mistakenly interpreted improved survival and increased detection with screening as evidence that screening saves lives. Few correctly recognized that only reduced mortality in a randomized trial constitutes evidence of the benefit of screening.[36] Improved survival rates and increased early detection do not necessarily prove that a cancer screening test saves lives. Nevertheless, these two statistics are often used to promote the benefits of screening.

If physicians are unclear about the worth of a cancer screening test, it is likely that the general public is probably unsure as well. Most people would want to know what their chance of dying from disease X is if they are screened compared to if they are not. Unfortunately, in some cases, we just do not have the answer. This dilemma is the focal point of the debate about breast cancer screening. The following chapters focus on the benefits and limitations of breast cancer screening and try to explain the crux of the debate about screening for this cancer.

American Cancer Society Guidelines for the Early Detection of Cancer

Cervical Cancer

- Cervical cancer testing should start at age 21, but women under age 21 should not be tested.

- Women between the ages of 21 and 29 should have a Pap test done every 3 years. HPV testing should not be used in this age group unless it's needed after an abnormal Pap test result.

- Women between the ages of 30 and 65 should have a Pap test plus an HPV test every 5 years. This is the preferred approach, but it's okay to have a Pap test alone every 3 years.

- Women over age 65 who have had regular cervical cancer testing in the past 10 years with normal results need not be tested for cervical cancer.

- Women with a history of cervical pre-cancer should continue to be tested for at least 20 years after that diagnosis, even if testing goes past age 65.

- Woman who have had a total hysterectomy for reasons not related to cervical cancer and who have no history of cervical cancer or serious pre-cancer need not be tested.

NOTE: All women who have been vaccinated against HPV should still follow the screening recommendations for their age groups.

Colorectal Cancer

- Regular screening should begin at age 45 for those at average risk for colorectal cancer and should continue to age 75.
- Those ages 76 through 85 should talk with their health care provider about whether continuing to get screened is appropriate.
- Those over age 85 should no longer get colorectal cancer screening.
- Colorectal cancer is a slow-growing cancer hence having a colonoscopy within 5 years provides little benefit. Most individuals (except those at high risk of developing this cancer) need to be screened once every 10 years.

NOTE: Those screened by tests other than colonoscopy, and if any abnormal findings are found, should have a colonoscopy.

Lung Cancer

- Those aged 55 to 74 who currently smoke or have quit smoking in the past 15 years or had at least a 30 pack-year smoking history should have yearly lung cancer screening with a low-dose CT scan (LDCT).

Prostate Cancer

- The American Cancer Society recommends that men make an informed decision with a health care provider about whether to be tested for prostate cancer. Research has not yet proven that the potential benefits of testing outweigh the harms of testing and treatment.

Source: American Cancer Society Guidelines for the Early Detection of Cancer. https://www.cancer.org/healthy/find-cancer-early/cancer-screening-guidelines/american-cancer-society-guidelines-for-the-early-detection-of-cancer.html. Reprinted by permission of the American Cancer Society, Inc. www.cancer.org. All rights reserved.

CHAPTER FIVE

Advances in Breast Cancer Detection: What Are the Options?

Medical research and technological advances in the area of breast cancer detection, diagnosis, and treatment have led to new medical, radiological, and surgical techniques designed to provide care to women with breast disease. Advances in breast cancer detection technology include new, safer ways to image the breast that do not include radiation exposure. In the early days of screening for breast cancer by mammography (i.e., the 1960s and 1970s), for example, the radiation dose was very high (10 to 35 rad) compared with current levels (0.2 rad). Also, new detection strategies aimed at finding distinctive "molecular signatures" of a premalignant or malignant breast tumor have the potential to revolutionize the detection and treatment of diseases.

Evidence clearly has shown that less-disfiguring surgical procedures, such as a lumpectomy, are equally good as, if not superior to, the radical mastectomy. With a lumpectomy, much of the breast and chest architecture is preserved. In this chapter, we examine the major breast imaging options available. However, given that technology changes rapidly, it is important to understand that some of the material considered cutting edge today may be out of date a year or more from now. Conversely, some of the material that is considered "experimental" today may become the norm a year or more from now.

Seeing Is Believing: Breast Screening Options

Before the use of mammography, early diagnosis of breast cancer was limited to a physician palpating the breast and looking for physical signs such as retraction or inversion of the nipples. With the discovery of x-rays by Wilhelm Conrad Roentgen in the late 19th century, x-rays were commonly used in the diagnosis and treatment of cancer. Mammography is essentially an x-ray procedure.

The development of mammography has a rich history spanning over 100 years. In 1913, Berlin surgeon Dr. Albert Salomon conducted a roentgeno-histological study on 3,000 mastectomies.[1] Using radiography of mastectomy specimens to demonstrate the spread of tumors to the axillary lymph nodes, he found microcalcifications (small calcium deposits that look like white specks on a mammogram) in x-ray images of tumor samples. Microcalcifications are usually benign, but they can be a sign of breast cancer if they appear in certain patterns and are clustered together, indicating a sign of precancerous cells or early breast cancer. Salomon's work provided substantial information about the pathological differences between cancerous and normal tissues. However, in this early mammography prototype, it was difficult to detect cancerous tissue in the breast because the tissue varied so much and the image quality was poor. Also, the dose of radiation was high.

In the early 1930s, Dr. Walter Vogel reported a radiographic classification of benign breast lesions and how the benign lesions were different from malignant lesions. At the same time, Dr. Paul S. Seabold presented his findings of radiographic diagnosis of breast disease. However, there still needed to be substantial improvement in the imaging technology, and despite Dr. Salomon, Dr. Vogel, Dr. Seabold, and others' research, use of mammography did not become common practice for decades.

In the mid-20th century, Dr. Gershon-Cohen and his colleague Dr. Helen Ingleby were lonely voices in claiming that mammography could help detect breast cancers that could not be discovered on physical examination. Yet, surgeons remained highly skeptical of mammography, and not helping matters, the images on mammography were still dark and hazy, and the radiation remained high. In 1949, Dr. Raul Leborgne, a pioneer in the enhancement of imaging quality, discovered that by compressing the breast before imaging, the x-ray could pick up small areas of calcification. He initiated imaging quality enhancement and emphasized differential diagnosis between benign and malignant calcifications.[2]

Prior to the 1960s, there was not much discussion about what mammography was and what it could do despite the technological advances being made. Women did not have a mammogram done because physicians did not routinely recommend that they should. Things changed, however, in the latter half of the 20th century with substantial advances made in mammographic techniques. In 1962, Dr. Robert Egan, using special films developed by Kodak, was able to diagnose 53 cases of occult breast cancer on mammography on a sample of 2,000 mammograms.[3] The images were more clear than was the case with early mammography and therefore easier to interpret. Egan's work presented data that strongly suggested the value of mammography in diagnosing breast cancer, and he showed that acceptable quality could be attained. Most importantly, mammography could enable differentiation between benign and malignant lesions. The ensuing widespread use of mammography is primarily attributed to the work of Dr. Egan.

The first compression mammography machine, an improvement on Leborgne's work, was developed in 1966. This machine pressed down on the breast tissue to enable better visualization of microcalcifications and tumors. With further advances in technology, screen-film mammography, and with machines that reduced radiation doses, mammography in the 1970s allowed for a high degree of accuracy to differentiate between benign and malignant disease, making it more feasible for x-ray mammography to be widely used in breast imaging. Based on the work of these early pioneers, the American College of Radiology (ACR) established committees and centers for mammography training on a countrywide level. In the 1960s, mammography became a subspecialty within radiology, and radiologists acquired substantial expertise in taking and reading breast x-rays. By the 1970s, clinics and hospitals in the United States were providing this service. In 1976, the American Cancer Society recommended that mammograms should be used as a screening tool for breast cancer.

Major improvements in the mammography equipment continued in partnership with industry and radiology, which led to further reduction in radiation dosage and improved clarity in imaging. Mammography was shown to be able to detect small breast cancers, which led to surgeons performing diagnostic biopsies, and experienced mammographers became adept at looking for suspicious signs that might indicate that cancer was present. In the latter half of the 20th century, mammography was viewed as an excellent means to detect early-stage breast cancer and, with that, an acknowledgment and acceptance of the potential benefits of mammography population-based screening by physicians and women. Mammography became the gold standard for screening for breast cancer in asymptomatic women.

Mammography is also used as a diagnostic tool to diagnose suspicious breast changes such as a lump, thickening, or nipple discharge. To clarify the difference between a screening test and a diagnostic test, screening tests are offered to asymptomatic people—we don't know who might have the disease. The screening test, which is not a diagnostic test, identifies individuals who should have further testing (e.g., diagnostic testing)—because they test positive on screening. A diagnostic test would serve to rule in or rule out disease and would provide a definitive result (yes, the disease is present or no, the disease is not present). Since the focus of this book is screening mammography, diagnostic mammography will not be discussed.

Mammography: Sensitivity and Specificity Issues

There are limitations to mammography, however. Mammography is not 100% accurate and is dependent on the skill of the radiologist reading the film, among other factors that will be explained later. It is technically one of the most difficult radiographic investigations to interpret. Finding a tumor is not always easy, as a cancerous lesion can be seen on a mammogram only if it looks different from surrounding breast tissue. In some cases, the cancer is indistinguishable from normal tissue. Hence, it is important to understand that negative findings on a mammogram do not always rule out breast cancer, and positive findings do not always indicate a malignancy. Readings vary depending on the age of the woman, breast density, positioning of the patient, time of her menstrual cycle, and skills of the radiologist in reading the film. Physician variability in reading the films has been well documented. Also, estimates of sensitivity (ability of a test to correctly identify those with the disease—true positive rate) and specificity (ability of the test to correctly identify those without the disease—true negative rate) of mammography will vary with the methods used to calculate these rates.

The overall sensitivity of screening mammography ranges from 71 to 92%. This wide range reflects the differences in mammography's ability to detect cancer when it is present. Among women older than age 50, the sensitivity ranges between 85 and 90%; however, sensitivity is lower among women younger than age 50 primarily because younger women tend to have denser breasts, making it more difficult to detect tumors on film. While overall the sensitivity is fairly high, which should be reassuring to women, the specificity is lower. Ranges of specificity have been shown to be between 30 and 65%. This implies that mammography is not always able to correctly identify those who do not have tumors. The specificity among younger women is not as good as that for women over age 50.

The debate among epidemiologists, oncologists, and radiologists is whether it is better to have a test that has a high sensitivity or one that has a high specificity. There is a trade-off. If the test has a high sensitivity, there is great comfort in knowing that a cancer will be found, if it exists (e.g., true positive). If a test has a high specificity, there is great comfort in knowing that cancer does not exist and will not be interpreted as being present (e.g., true negative). But what are the implications of a false positive test result or, for that matter, a false negative test result? False positive test results mean that the test was read as showing disease when in fact there is none. False negative test results mean that the test was read as negative—no disease—when in fact disease is present. With a false positive result, an individual will undergo additional tests to definitively rule in or rule out disease. Some of these tests are invasive, they are costly, and the anxiety of thinking that cancer is present can be very upsetting. With a false negative result, an individual is given a false sense of security—I am disease-free. What a relief. There would be no follow-up and no further testing, yet the disease is indeed present and could progress to a more advanced stage in the absence of treatment.

A large-scale 10-year study based on 9,762 screening mammograms and 10,905 screening clinical breast examinations performed by a physician found that of the women screened by mammography, one-quarter had at least one false positive mammogram reading, 13.4% had at least one false positive clinical breast examination, and 31.7% had at least one false positive result for either test. Among women who did not have breast cancer, an estimated 19% had to have a biopsy after 10 mammograms compared to only 6.2% after 10 clinical breast exams. Over 10 years, one-third of the women screened had abnormal test results requiring additional evaluation, even though no breast cancer was present.[4] What this all means is that screening for breast cancer either by mammography or by clinical breast exam is not precise and that false positive results are not uncommon.

The good news is that the more films a radiologist interprets, the greater the likelihood that his or her skills will improve. Volume is an important factor in honing skills. Low-volume radiologists and medium-volume radiologists have lower sensitivity rates than high-volume radiologists.[5] Reader volume is a very important component and determinant of mammogram sensitivity and specificity.

The not-so-good news is that the more mammograms a woman has over time, the greater the likelihood of a false positive reading. If a 40-year-old woman has annual screenings by mammogram over the course of 10 years, she would have a 30% chance of having at least one abnormal screening examination that would require a diagnostic workup, a 28% chance of at least one false positive exam, and a 7.5% chance of having a breast biopsy performed. Alternatively, a 50-year-old woman having the same 10 mammograms over 10 years has a 26% chance of at least one abnormal screening exam, a 23% chance of having at least one false positive exam, and a 10.4% chance of having at least one breast biopsy.[6]

While the proportion of false positive readings is only a small number of the total number of mammograms performed, it should be understood that the probability increases by age. However, the overwhelming majority of false positive readings actually turn out to be false alarms. For example, among 100 women aged 40 to 49 who have an abnormal mammogram result, 94 will not have cancer. But these women would have had to undergo further testing before a breast cancer diagnosis could be ruled out. The financial and emotional burden of false positive readings could be significant.

Balancing Mammography's Potential Benefits and Potential Harms

So which is preferable? Is it "better" for a screening test to have a high sensitivity (e.g., high percentage of true positives) or a high specificity (e.g., low percentage of false positives)? Ideally, a screening test should be both highly sensitive and highly specific. But, in reality, this is not the case with mammography. It is not 100% accurate, unfortunately, which raises the question: To what extent does mammography screening increase the likelihood that a true cancer would be detected? Some cancers are so slow growing that failure to detect them would not make a difference in overall survival (e.g., DCIS), which brings up the issue of overdiagnosis (i.e., tumors detected on screening that never would have led to clinical symptoms).

Overdiagnosis, or overdetection, in cancer screening is defined as the detection of cancers that grow so slowly that they are unlikely to be diagnosed during a person's lifetime and would not cause the individual any harm in the absence of screening.[7] That is, these cancers, if never diagnosed, would not cause harm if a woman had not been screened. There is considerable debate both in the United States and in other countries about the "value" of mammography screening. Does overdiagnosis weaken the potential benefits of population-based screening? Overdiagnosis is acknowledged as one of the most serious downsides of population breast screening; yet the extent to which screening "causes" overdiagnosis is an unresolved issue at this time. We know it exists, but to what extent is a question that is difficult to answer.

Estimates of the prevalence of overdiagnosis are highly variable. A 2007 systematic review of the literature found an extremely broad range of overdiagnosis estimates—ranging from 0 to 62%!—and also highlighted that source (primary) studies were prone to biases that may have served to over- or underestimate the magnitude of breast cancer overdiagnosis.[8] Yet, another systematic review reported an overdiagnosis rate of 6.5% with a range from 1 to 10%.[9] In reality, overdiagnosis rates will differ among different types of study design (randomized clinical trial, cohort study, etc.) and who is included in the study (study sample characteristics).

Researchers using 1975 through 2012 data from the Surveillance, Epidemiology, and End Results (SEER) program looked at the issue of tumor size and overdiagnosis from mammography screening.[10] Since one of the goals of screening mammography is to detect small asymptomatic, cancerous tumors before they grow large, the researchers posited that effective screening should lead to the detection of a larger number of small tumors and fewer large tumors over time. Their analysis showed that after the widespread use of mammography, the proportion of detected breast tumors that were small (<2 cm or in situ carcinomas) increased from 36 to 68% over the study time period. The proportion of detected tumors that were large (>2 cm) decreased from 64 to 32%. What this implies is that these results were due less to a decrease in the incidence of large tumors and more to the result of a substantial increase in the detection of small tumors. The researchers calculated that only 30 of the 162 additional small tumors per 100,000 women that were diagnosed were expected to progress to become large, and the remaining 132 cases per 100,000 women were overdiagnosed.

A 2017 major study, conducted by researchers at the Nordic Cochrane Centre in collaboration with researchers from Norway, looked into the effects of breast cancer screening programs and found a high risk of overdiagnosis, which raised doubts about screening benefits.[11] Based on the analysis of the data, the researchers concluded that breast cancer screening was not associated with a reduction in the incidence of advanced cancer and that one in three breast cancers detected in women offered screening are likely overdiagnosed. Their findings support previous findings from the Cochrane review of screening for breast cancer with mammography that examined the high risk of overtreating women.[12] A subsequent chapter will discuss this in much more detail.

The fact is that many factors contribute to the variability in reported estimates of breast cancer overdiagnosis, including but not limited to lack of agreement on the definition of overdiagnosis; disagreement on what constitutes the denominator for calculating overdiagnosis; disagreement on including DCIS or invasive cancer, or both; disagreement on the timeframe to measure overdiagnosis; and framing of the extent of overdiagnosis (relative or absolute estimates). It is important to raise the issue not to make women scared of having a mammogram or other breast screening modalities, rather to make women aware that it exists and understand the potential consequences such as unnecessary biopsies, breast surgery, and treatment. Advances in precision and accuracy of screening technology are helping to permit a more precise diagnosis of suspicious breast lesions, which hopefully will reduce the uncertainty in diagnosing breast disease.

Suffice it to say, the issue is complicated and continues to be a source of debate among breast cancer researchers. There remains a need for more systematic evaluation of the extent of overdiagnosis relative to screening benefit and the burden of overtreatment.

Ensuring Quality Standards

Although mammography is not a perfect screening tool, it remains a highly effective method for early breast cancer detection. Weighing the balance of benefits to harms, overall getting screened is probably better than foregoing screening. Yes, there are debates about the extent of overdiagnosis as well as the overall value of mammography (which will be discussed in the next chapter), but, despite the limitations, mammography is considered to be a valued tool in detecting cancer at an early stage. One important factor in ensuring the efficacy of mammography is to maintain high quality standards regarding the safety of the units.

Prior to 1992, there were neither uniform standards to ensure that mammography was safe and reliable nor uniform standards for technicians and for physicians who read the film. In the United States, states had varying quality control standards that resulted in inconsistent and nonuniform readings. There were no record systems that could provide reliable and comprehensive data to permit the evaluation of the performance of screening mammography.

In an effort to set basic minimum national standards, Congress enacted the Mammography Quality Standards Act of 1992 (MQSA). This act provided federal uniform quality control standards, instituted a system of inspection of mammography clinics, and set training standards for technicians who perform mammography tests as well as for physicians who read mammography x-rays. It further required that women receive direct written notification of their test results. The act further stipulated that the FDA be responsible for accrediting and inspecting mammography facilities to certify that each meets MQSA standards. Every facility is required to prominently display their FDA certificate.

A section of the MQSA authorized the establishment of a breast cancer screening surveillance system. In 1994, the Department of Health and Human Services was authorized to fund through the National Cancer Institute the Breast Cancer Surveillance Consortium (BCSC), which develops and conducts collaborative research projects that use common data elements contributed by its network of seven mammography registries across the United States. The BCSC evaluates the performance of mammography in community practice and related screening and breast cancer outcomes, and today it is a national resource for population-based research on breast cancer. To date, the Consortium has collected data for more than 1.5 million women and 4 million mammograms.

In 1999, a revised ruling designed to strengthen standards relating to equipment so as to ensure that each unit is capable of producing high-quality mammograms took effect. The revised MQSA also required that mobile units be checked for acceptable performance each time the unit is moved to a new location and before any examinations are performed.[13] As of 2001, there were over 9,600 MQSA-certified mammography facilities in the United States and its territories.

While it is important to ensure the quality and safety of the mammography machine, it is equally important to ensure that mammograms are read and interpreted in a uniform way. That being said, radiologists' accuracy of interpreting mammograms vary. Those who read more mammograms have better accuracy than those who read fewer films. Clearly the number of years of experience reading mammograms affect accuracy. Also, radiologists who only specialize in reading mammogram films have higher accuracy rates than those who read films less frequently. Going to the same facility where previous films are stored helps because the radiologist could compare prior films to the current one. Complicating matters, however, is the fact that clinical characteristics of a woman can affect accuracy. As has been stated numerous times in this chapter, dense breasts are more difficult to read on image than fatty breasts. Women who have breast implants and women who have breast scarring also present a challenge to the radiologist.

There are occasional reports of shoddy mammography clinics in which either the quality of the film is poor or the interpretation of the film is substandard. In each of the last five years, more than 40% of the mammography facilities in the United States were cited for violating one or more federal rules! While inspections are done primarily by the individual states, follow-up varies tremendously. The FDA can levy fines of up to $10,000 a day to facilities in violation of federal rules, although it rarely does so. Clearly, those agencies that oversee the quality and safety of mammography facilities need to become more aggressive in their duty.

Advances in Breast Imaging

In the recent past, women whose mammograms looked suspicious or abnormal had few follow-up options available. They were often instructed to return within six months for a follow-up mammogram, but this "wait and see" approach not only increases the anxiety of uncertainty but also could jeopardize early treatment, possibly lowering the chance for survival if a malignant lesion is detected later. Detecting a cancer before it has spread to other parts of the body is the objective and purpose of screening. Improving the means for early detection, of course, would be in the best interest of the patient.

Over the past two decades, there have been exciting advances in breast cancer detection technology, including new ways to image the breast and new detection strategies aimed at finding distinctive "molecular signatures" of a premalignant or malignant breast tumor. Several highly sophisticated technologies now permit a more precise way to detect early tumors and lesions. The following presents a brief description of some of these tools.

Contrast-enhanced mammography (CEM) is a breast imaging technique in which a contrast agent is given intravenously to allow a stronger contrast between a breast tumor and the surrounding tissue. While not a tool for everyone, CEM may be useful in addition to mammography in women who are at higher-than-average risk of breast cancer who are not recommended for breast MRI (such as women with dense breasts) or who cannot have breast MRI.

Digital mammography and digital breast tomosynthesis is used as an adjunct to screen-film mammography. This technology can detect tumors that are not visible on mammography. Whereas screen-film mammography uses x-ray equipment to record images, digital mammography uses more specialized computerized equipment to capture a digital image and delivers lower doses of radiation. Digital mammography, which received FDA approval in 2000, uses x-rays to create an image of the breast on a computer screen. A detector responds to x-ray exposure and sends an electronic signal to a computer to be digitized and processed. Computer programs aid in the detection and characterization of breast masses and calcifications that allow the radiologist to adjust images to help detect subtle differences between tissues. The images can be stored and retrieved electronically. There is no film to develop. Digital mammograms often take more views of each breast, but they use less radiation than film mammography probably because smaller areas of the breast are imaged in each view.

Digital mammography offers advantages over conventional mammography in that the digital image can be manipulated postprocessing; adjustments in brightness and contrast are possible, and selected areas of the breast can be electronically magnified. In theory, this could help the radiologist better detect tumors obscured by dense beast tissue frequently seen in younger women. Digital mammograms rely on computer-aided detection (CAD) systems, which use the computer to highlight suspicious areas for more intense review, perhaps reducing the number of false positive results. This technique is particularly useful in cases that would ordinarily require a second reader because of suspicious findings. The CAD system is designed to assist the radiologist in also reducing the number of negative readings by focusing attention on areas that might warrant a second review. However, CAD used alone has very low specificity, and while digital mammography has the ability to "see" more than conventional mammography, there are limitations, including the cost of the test.

How much better is digital mammography compared to film mammography? A large clinical trial, the Digital Mammographic Imaging Screening Trial (DMIST), analyzed data on 46,720 asymptomatic women who presented for screening mammography at 33 sites in the United States and Canada. All underwent both digital and film mammography.[14] Results showed that digital mammography was significantly better than conventional film mammography at detecting breast cancer in young women, premenopausal and perimenopausal women, and women with dense breasts. Film mammography tended to perform better in women aged 65 years or older with fatty breasts, but this result was not statistically significant. Given the findings from numerous studies showing the superiority of digital mammography over film mammography, digital mammography has largely replaced film mammography as the preferred means of screening for breast cancer.

While nearly all cancers will be apparent in fatty breasts, only half will be visible in extremely dense breasts.[15] A new technique, *digital breast tomosynthesis (DBT)*, or 3D mammography, promises to improve detection of tumors in women with dense breasts. DBT was approved by the FDA in 2011 and is a relatively new technique for breast imaging that relies on the construction of a 3D image of the breast with multiple high-resolution x-rays. The images are synthesized by a computer to form a 3D image. The 3D image sets serve to minimize the tissue overlap that can hide cancers or make it difficult to distinguish normal overlapping breast tissue from tumors. It is important to note that DBT uses low-dose x-rays and can be used in combination with the standard mammogram technology (e.g., 2D imaging).

While DBT detects 40% more breast cancers than traditional 2D mammography, it will also find more benign lesions.[16] At this time, it should not serve as a replacement for population-based mammography screening. However, it could be very useful for screening high-risk individuals (e.g., those with a family history of breast cancer, dense breasts, younger than age 50) and can also be used as a diagnostic tool for women experiencing symptoms such as a lump, pain, skin dimpling, or nipple discharge. For example, DBT-guided core needle biopsy capability is useful for suspicious lesions seen only on DBT.

Of the few studies that have been done on DBT, findings show good patient and physician acceptance, very good sensitivity, and improvement in breast characterization.[17,18] One large-scale study found that screening with DBT is associated with increased specificity and an increased proportion of breast cancers detected with better prognosis compared with 2D digital mammography. In the subgroup of women aged 40 to 49 years with non-dense breasts, the cancer detection rate using DBT was 1.7 per 1,000 women higher compared with the rate using 2D digital mammography. Among women with dense breasts, the cancer detection rate was 2.27 per 1,000 women higher for DBT.[19] There are no clinical trials of DBT as of this writing.

Of particular interest is whether DBT should replace conventional mammographic views or should be an adjunct to mammography or some combination of the two. We know that variability in mammographic interpretation is a major weak link in the assessment of mammographic images. Given the complexity of DBT, special training for radiologists will be needed. Also, the cost of this test must be factored into the decision-making. DBT may not be fully covered by some health insurance plans. That being said, DBT is rapidly emerging as an important new imaging tool and is viewed by radiologists as another significant advance in mammography technology.

Magnetic resonance imaging (MRI) of the breast is another means for screening women who are at increased risk for breast cancer. Breast MRI uses radio waves and strong magnets to create very detailed, cross-sectional 3D images of the breast. It does not use x-rays; rather a magnet is linked to a computer to show detailed images of areas in the body without the use of radiation.

The test generates an image by measuring the responses of tissue components to a magnetic field. A nonradioactive contrast agent is injected into a vein to improve the clarity of detailed images of the breast tissue. MRI of the breast can be effective for women with dense breasts and for women with breast implants (e.g., to detect leaks or ruptures) and can be used after breast cancer is detected by other means to determine the extent of the tumor. MRI can be used as well to diagnose fibroadenoma, a benign breast tumor most common among women younger than age 30.

A 2019 multicenter, randomized controlled trial of 40,373 Dutch women between the ages of 50 and 75 years provided much-needed evidence that MRI of the breast is highly effective at finding cancerous tumors among women with dense breasts.[20] The primary outcome of this study was the incidence of interval cancers during a two-year screening period. The study provides strong evidence that getting a MRI after mammogram was much more effective in finding tumors than mammogram alone in women with very dense breasts. What the study could not tell us is whether mammogram plus MRI reduces breast cancer deaths. The answer to this question will take years to be determined.

Although MRI can find some cancers not seen on a mammogram, it has a higher false positive rate than other forms of mammography, and it does not detect microcalcifications well. Hence, breast MRI should not be used for population-based screening; rather it should be used as an addition to mammography for women at high lifetime risk of breast cancer, for women with breast implants, and perhaps for high-risk women under age 40. Women who are at moderate increased risk should talk with their physician about MRI screening. Women who are not considered to be at risk for breast cancer probably should not have a MRI of the breast.[21] Although more costly than other types of mammography (an average MRI of the breast costs approximately $1,000 versus $100 for screening mammography), most major insurance companies will cover some of the costs if the woman is considered to be high risk.

There are several other tests that are used to investigate suspicious lesions in the breast. These are not considered to be useful for population-based screening, but are most helpful in detecting abnormalities in high-risk women. They are adjuncts to mammography, not replacements. *Breast ultrasound* uses high-frequency sound waves to generate an image. Used as a diagnostic tool, ultrasound is used to further investigate suspicious findings from a mammogram (e.g., a mass that could be a solid tissue or a harmless cyst containing fluid). Ultrasound imaging devices emit high-frequency sound waves and generate distinctive echoes that a computer uses to generate an image (e.g., sonogram). A fluid-filled cyst has a different sound than a solid mass.

There are two types of ultrasound: handheld and automated whole-breast ultrasound. Handheld ultrasound is operator dependent; the radiologist must rely only on the representative images obtained by the technologist. In automated whole-breast ultrasound (ABUS), the entirety of the breast can be imaged and reviewed by the radiologist, which allows for more reliable and reproducible imaging of the entirety of the breast and more extensive images for annual comparison. It also allows the radiologist to interpret the entire data set as opposed to representative images obtained by a technologist.[22] A newer technology, the addition of computer-aided detection (CAD) software for ABUS, has the potential to improve the screening performance of radiologists by improving the efficiency of reading the images and has a faster scan time compared to handheld ultrasound. However, the cost of ABUS has to be taken into account.

Ultrasound imaging of the breast is highly sensitive in detecting tumors in women with dense breasts, which is a good thing because cancers detected in women with dense breasts are larger and more often node positive. Further, ultrasound can distinguish between solid tumors and fluid-filled cysts. Studies have shown that ultrasound significantly increases detection of small, largely invasive, node-negative cancers.[23] While breast ultrasound also can be used to evaluate lumps that are hard to see on a mammogram, this test does not detect microcalcifications well, nor can it detect small tumors less than 5 mm. As such, ultrasound is used as a follow-up to a suspicious mammogram and as part of other diagnostic procedures such as fine-needle aspiration or needle biopsy. However, it is not a test that would be used, or should be used, on the general population. It is best used on women with dense breasts who are at high risk of developing breast cancer. It should be used as an adjunct to mammography.

Other Imaging Technologies

There are other, high-tech means now being used to detect breast cancer, but none are considered suitable for population-based screening. Some rely on radioactive compounds, while others aim to identify cancerous tissue by analyzing temperature. *Digital infrared imaging (DII), or breast thermography,* approved by the FDA in 1982 as a breast imaging procedure to be used in addition to other imaging tests and/or examination procedures, is based on the principle that metabolic activity and vascular circulation in both precancerous tissue and the area surrounding a developing breast cancer is almost always higher than in normal breast tissue.[24] While mammography, ultrasound, MRI, and other imaging tools rely primarily on finding the physical tumor, DII detects the heat produced by increased blood vessel circulation based on images of temperature variations. Temperature variations are thought to be very early signs of breast cancer or precancer, and studies have shown that an abnormal infrared image is the single most important early warning for developing breast cancer.

DII involves no radiation, compression of the breast, or intravenous contrast, and its sensitivity and specificity are estimated to be 90%; however, DII does not identify microcalcifications,[25] nor does it have the ability to pinpoint the location of a tumor. As such, it should be used in combination with, not instead of, mammography or other imaging tools. DII has only been cleared by the FDA as an "adjunctive" tool—meaning for use alongside a primary test like mammography. It is a very sophisticated technology and requires expertise to interpret the infrared images.

Molecular breast imaging (MBI) is a new means of imaging the breast. Approved for use in 1999 by the FDA, the objective of MBI is to detect molecular markers for breast cancer, focusing on genetic damage/genetic changes. Molecular markers could identify women who should undergo more frequent screening or who might benefit from newer imaging technologies to monitor changes in the breast tissue. MBI relies on nuclear medicine in which a short-term radioactive agent (a tracer) is administered intravenously and absorbed into tissues. A special camera (a nuclear medicine scanner or gamma camera) records the activity of a radioactive tracer. Normal tissue and cancerous tissue react differently to the tracer, which is seen in the images produced by the gamma camera. Breast cancer cells appear to absorb more of the tracer than do healthy cells. Tumors will light up—the radiologist will see a "hot spot" on the camera. The breast is not compressed as it is in conventional mammography, allowing for a 3D view. MBI's accuracy rate in detecting breast cancer is over 90%, which is higher than mammography's 84%. One potential drawback is that it exposes the whole body to radiation, not just the breast.

Positron emission mammography (PEM) is another newer imaging test of the breast. Similar to a PET scan (positron emission tomography), the PEM scan is designed to detect small clusters of cancer cells in the breast. A form of sugar attached to a radioactive particle is injected into the blood to detect cancer cells. Cancer cells tend to consume more sugar than normal cells, and this can help identify tumors. As with MBI, PEM exposes the whole body to radiation.

Senographe Pristina Mammography System, developed and designed by female engineers and designers at GE, is a 3D digital breast tomosynthesis system that provides high diagnostic accuracy at low radiation exposure. Traditional mammography systems compress the breast automatically. This system allows women to control the compression during mammography by means of a wireless remote control device. That is, women can adjust the compression after the breast is positioned by the technician to set the compression to a force that feels right for her. By being able to control the compression force, a woman is in control of the system and can feel more comfortable during the procedure. Many women dislike going for a mammogram because of the pain and discomfort. The system is designed to ensure that the woman is more comfortable. A study conducted on 160 patients who used the patient-assisted compression across two sites in Europe found high levels of satisfaction.[26] A clinical trial comparing this system to the traditional system by assessing patient experience related to discomfort is estimated to be completed by end of 2020.

Image-Guided Techniques

There are a variety of image-guided procedures used to supplement mammography, the objective of which is to lead to more accurate characterization of breast masses and less surgery for breast cancer patients. Image-guided core-needle breast biopsy, for example, involves a stereotactic or ultrasound-guided procedure to permit the precise location of the abnormal tissue seen on mammogram. Stereotactic refers to the use of a computer and scanning device to create a 3D image. A stereotactic needle biopsy guided by mammography is actually less expensive and less invasive than a traditional surgical excisional biopsy and results in less breast deformity. More information about this technique will be provided in the chapter on breast cancer treatment.

New technologies are on the horizon, including magnetic resonance elastography, electrical impedance spectroscopy, microwave imaging spectroscopy, and near infrared spectroscopic imaging. These are highly complex and sophisticated technologies that are intended to identify changes associated with tumor growth. These do not pose radiation risk, do not require compression of the breast, and, at this point in time, are not appropriate for population-based screening. However, they are not designed as first-line screening.

What about Low-Tech Options?

While the advances in sophisticated imaging devices have done much to increase the accuracy and precision of breast cancer diagnosis, there is clearly a role for low-tech screening. Not everyone can afford a mammogram. Mammography screening may not be available in some areas, especially in low- and middle-income countries. Two of the most important low-tech mechanisms for detecting abnormalities in the breast are breast self-exam (BSE) and clinical breast exam (CBE).

Although the American Cancer Society no longer recommends that all women perform monthly breast self-exams *per se*, every woman should know how to examine her own breasts. Learning how to examine one's breasts and becoming familiar with the lumps and bumps helps an individual to notice a change in the texture of her breasts. A BSE is best done several days after menstruation ends, a time when the breasts are less likely to be swollen and tender. It is important to stress that most breast lumps are not cancer. Many could be fluid-filled cysts that can be left alone or can be drained if they are too uncomfortable. A fibrous breast will feel lumpy, but for the most part, it is not cancerous.

Changes in the texture and size (thickening or swelling) and discharge from the nipple or puckering/dimpling around the nipple are signs that something is not right. Any breast change from the normal should be a cause for concern and should be discussed with your physician. The following diagram shows the correct way to perform a BSE. The self-exam can be done standing in the shower or lying down with a pillow under the shoulder. It is important to check all areas of the breast: the armpit to the collarbone, the breast itself, and the nipple area. Looking in a mirror helps visualize changes in shape, size, or skin texture. The BSE should be done in a circular manner, using three fingers (not the tips of the fingers, rather use the pads of the finger). Light, medium, and deep pressure should be applied. The right hand should be used to examine the left breast and the left hand should be used to examine the right breast.

The clinical breast exam should be done by a physician or other trained health professional. The exam includes an inspection of the breasts as well as palpation of the breast and chest area, including the lymph nodes above and below the collarbone and under each arm. Special attention is given to the shape and texture of the breasts, the location of any lumps, and the area around the armpits. It is often helpful if the CBE can be scheduled within the same month as the mammogram since a CBE can alert the physician to unusual lumps that should be investigated further by mammography. However, the CBE is no longer recommended for average-risk, asymptomatic women based on lack of clear benefits for CBE alone or even in conjunction with mammography.[27]

BSE and CBE are not substitutes for mammography. The sensitivity of CBE ranges from 48 to 69%, far lower than that for mammography. Also, a CBE cannot differentiate malignant from benign palpable lesions. Determining whether a lump is just a lump or whether it is more serious is the most challenging part of a CBE.

Concluding Thoughts/Take-Home Message

While no screening modality is 100% perfect, the accuracy, sensitivity, and specificity of the imaging technologies discussed herein have enabled women to seek care for a cancer that they may not have had any idea that they had. Yet, every test has its pros and cons, which hopefully have been discussed in this chapter. And none of the newer technologies have been shown to reduce the risk of dying from breast cancer, one of the tenets of screening. Perhaps some are too new and more studies are needed to quantify the extent to which mortality is reduced.

Because no single imaging device can accurately detect all types of breast abnormalities in different breast tissue, breast cancer screening should not necessarily be limited to one modality. Multiple imaging techniques are appropriate to detect and diagnose cancer in individuals who have a suspicious mammogram. Clearly, the more sophisticated devices are not appropriate for population-based screening, but they are very useful for women who, because of family history, age, dense breasts, and other factors, are considered to be at higher risk for developing breast cancer. In some instances, however, these highly sophisticated imaging tests might detect more tumors, some of which would be benign, resulting in too many false alarms. The focus now is on reducing the number of false positive test results, improving the detection of tumors in women with dense breasts, and continuing to reduce the amount of radiation to which a patient is exposed.

An interesting study (paid for by Google) looked at the use of artificial intelligence (AI) in radiology. Researchers from Google and medical centers in the United States and Britain compared the reading of mammography scans by AI and by radiologists.[28] Mammograms from 76,000 women in Britain and 15,000 women in the United States, whose diagnosis of breast cancer was already known, were read by AI and compared to the results from the radiologists who originally read the scans. In the U.S. scans, AI resulted in an almost 10% reduction in false negative readings (mammogram mistakenly read as normal but cancer was present) and about 6% reduction in false positives (the scan was read to be abnormal but actually no was cancer present). On the British mammograms, AI reduced false negatives by 3% and false positives by 1%. The takeaway point from this study is that AI can be more accurate than humans; however, the researchers said that it was not the intent of AI to replace radiologists! The AI tool, however, can be a valuable asset in enhancing human performance and flagging suspicious scans that would be further investigated by physicians.

Despite all the advancements, breast cancer screening and mammography are synonymous in the public's mind. Although it has its limitations, mammography remains the most cost-efficient, safe, and economic means of population-based screening for breast cancer. Mammography still remains the most effective mass screening technology presently available. Yet it is not without controversy. The following chapter discusses the results of large-scale breast cancer clinical trials and, in doing so, will underscore the doubts some have about the value of mammography.

CHAPTER SIX

Breast Cancer Screening Guidelines

The potential value of screening mammography has been examined in scores of studies and randomized clinical trials. The large-scale randomized trials that will be discussed in the next chapter differed in many ways, including study design, eligibility considerations, study population characteristics, interventions (screening protocols differed), study outcomes, duration of follow-up, and analysis of data. These differences make it difficult to compare and contrast findings and equally difficult to make recommendations about who should be screened, at what age, and how frequently. Although the overwhelming majority of women will not develop breast cancer in their lifetime (the risk of being diagnosed with breast cancer over the next 10 years for a 50-year-old cancer-free woman is just 2.3%[1]), the question remains: to what extent does mammography screening improve survival among those who test positive for breast cancer? Another important question is, Who would best benefit by mammography screening? Should women with higher risk factors for this cancer receive more frequent screening and start at an earlier age than those who do not have a high risk of developing breast cancer? While risk factors were presented in a previous chapter, this chapter focuses on key risk factors (i.e., age and race/ethnicity, sexual orientation, physically disabled) in more detail, as well as the implications for women regarding breast cancer screening.

From a policy perspective, there are many unanswered questions. Do the imperfections of the studies invalidate or negate the importance of their findings? Trend data show that over the past decades, breast cancer mortality has declined. Is this decline a result of better detection and treatment? For those whose cancer was detected at an early, more treatable stage, the answer would most probably be a resounding yes.

From a patient perspective, the perceived risk of breast cancer will differ among women. For some, mammogram screening is a way to "be sure" that everything is OK. Having an annual mammogram is considered to be the "best" way to "catch" cancer at an early stage. Peace of mind is something that cannot be discounted in the debate about the value of mammography. For others, ignorance is bliss: I feel fine, and I have no symptoms. Why should I bother with the discomfort and expense of a mammogram?

Certainly an individual's perspective on the benefits and harms of screening, as well as her age, ethnicity, personal values, and recommendations from her physician, will determine how often, if at all, she will schedule a mammogram. If a woman believes that she is at increased risk of developing breast cancer, the way she and her physician approach screening might be different from that among women who are not at high risk for breast cancer.

Understanding risk factors is important for many reasons, including how to formulate population-based breast cancer screening guidelines. Guidelines for disease screening are generally prepared for the general population; yet, those individuals with a higher risk for a disease need to be handled somewhat differently. For example, one would not implement a population-based screening test for sickle cell anemia because this disease is not prevalent in the general population. However, among a subset of the population (i.e., African Americans), sickle cell anemia is much more common, which implies that screening should be targeted to the high-risk group. Regarding breast cancer, age and ethnicity are important factors to consider when designing mammogram screening guidelines.

For many cancer screening programs, there is a relatively narrow age range in which screening is worthwhile. Since breast cancer is rare among very young women (i.e., younger than age 35) and among older women (i.e., over age 70), screening guidelines need to reflect this reality. If population-based screening was offered to all women over age 25 or 30 through age 79, for example, only a very small number would potentially benefit from screening, while a much larger number of women would potentially be harmed as a result of false positive readings. And, as was discussed previously, the cost of further testing to rule in or rule out breast cancer can be substantial. In human terms, there is no way to put a price on the anxiety and uncertainty a woman experiences as she waits for the pathology results. From an economic perspective, the benefits of screening all women regardless of age would probably not outweigh the costs.

Since we know that the incidence of breast cancer increases with age, the potential benefits of screening do outweigh the potential harms among older women (i.e., above age 50 but younger than age 70). That being said, the age at which mammography ceases to be beneficial is unclear.[2,3] Women over age

69, for example, probably would not realize the same benefits of screening as a woman aged 50 or 55. In older women, there are fewer years in which breast cancer could or would cause symptoms or death. There are competing factors such as heart disease, diabetes, and other chronic diseases that are much more likely to result in death before breast cancer would. Additionally, it is possible that a screening program for older women would detect cancers that would not be considered clinically important. That is, even if left alone, the cancer would not necessarily require testing or treatment, nor would it increase the risk of death from the cancer.

Breast Cancer Screening Guidelines for the Younger Woman

Discussion about whether to offer mammogram screening to specific age cohorts is difficult, complex, and emotional. The debate about the potential magnitude of the benefit of screening mammography for women younger than age 50 is especially contentious. What is the incremental benefit of beginning screening at age 40 or age 45 rather than at age 50? The answer is not clear cut. Women in their 40s are biologically different from those in their 50s and 60s. In particular, mammograms done on premenopausal women in their 40s are more difficult to interpret. Among this cohort, there are more false positive readings, which would trigger diagnostic testing. The overwhelming majority of these women end up not having cancer, but the anxiety, cost, and discomfort of undergoing additional testing must be considered. Also, there are more false negative readings among this cohort compared to women over age 50.

If one tries to glean answers from the findings from the eight randomized clinical trials and meta-analyses, the general consensus is that overall, the results are mixed. Australian researchers reviewed the evidence about the value of mammography screening for women between the ages of 40 and 49 years, and they concluded that approximately 2,600 women would be needed to be screened to prevent 1 death from breast cancer 13 years later.[4] If one applied their estimates to a hypothetical cohort of 10,000 women who were offered screening every 2 years beginning at age 40 instead of age 50, the expected benefit would be a saving of 7 lives after 13 years. I am not a betting woman, but these odds are not very compelling in my opinion.

Taking this example one step further, of the 10,000 women who received screening, 2,000 would in all likelihood have an abnormal mammogram that would require additional testing. Two hundred thirty of the 2,000 women would have a biopsy performed, of which 100 invasive cancers would be found. Twenty-one would end up being diagnosed with ductal carcinoma in situ (DCIS), and since the current thinking is that DCIS is best left alone, screening would not necessarily have been beneficial for these women. Based on these estimates, the overwhelming majority of the original 10,000 women would not end up having breast cancer.

The Australian model assumes that the 40 to 49 age group is homogeneous. But it could be argued that the benefit of screening would be greater in the 45 to 49 year-old group as compared to the 40 to 44 year-old group. The likelihood of finding more breast cancers in the 45 to 49 year-old cohort is probably greater than in the 40 to 44 year-old cohort given what we know about the epidemiology of breast cancer. Breast cancer is still rare among women younger than age 45, and this must be taken into consideration when formulating breast cancer screening guidelines.

Age, of course, is not the only risk factor for breast cancer. Women with a family history would probably benefit by earlier screening, but making recommendations on an individual basis is not the same as making recommendations for the larger population. Those who are at higher risk for developing breast cancer should not be considered the same as women who are not considered to be at risk based on their personal characteristics.

The preceding discussion raises an interesting issue of screening for breast cancer based on age (i.e., age-based breast cancer screening) or risk (i.e., risk-based breast cancer screening). Would screening based on risk yield better results than screening based on age? At present, all mammography screening programs use an age-based rather than a risk-based protocol. In order to test whether one approach would be better than the other, a study was conducted to test the hypothesis that risk-based screening will reduce both short-term benefits and harms compared to age-based screening.[5]

The study compared two approaches to screening women in their 40s: one was an age-based approach to screening all women each year beginning at age 45 years and the other was a risk-based screening of higher-risk women aged 40 to 49. The risk-based approach was intended to balance the benefits (i.e., early cancer detection) with the harms (i.e., false positive results, overdiagnosis, anxiety). Primary outcome variables were number of cancers detected, false positive mammograms, and benign biopsy results. The findings showed that age-based screening beginning at age 45 detected more cancers than the risk-based approach but resulted in more false positive mammograms and benign biopsy results. Risk-based screening yielded fewer mammograms and detected only 1 of 16 screening-detectable cancers. The risk-based approach exposed more women to delays in diagnosis; however, there were fewer false positive mammograms and benign biopsy results. This study showed that 75 to 80% of screening-detectable cancers in the 40 to 49 year-old age group would be missed by using the risk-based screening approach.[6,7]

Because the detectable preclinical phase for breast cancer is shorter in younger women who develop breast cancer compared with those in women 50 years and older, a key issue is deciding on an appropriate screening interval. Should there be annual screening? Biannual screening? The National

Cancer Institute (NCI) suggests that women in their 40s get screened every one to two years, depending on individual risk factors.[8] This sounds like the NCI is hedging its bets. The problem is that there are not good data from which recommendations could be made. And that is the crux of the problem. Given the paucity of data, the most prudent course of action is for the individual to decide for herself, in consultation with her physician, whether and at what age to initiate mammogram screening. It sounds as if I am hedging my bets as well.

The current debate about mammography guidelines makes it sound like an either/or decision, but the issue is more complex, more nuanced, than that. The cutoff of age 50 is somewhat arbitrary. How does one differentiate a 45-year old woman from a 51-year old woman? The body of evidence shows that there is a benefit of mammography screening for women aged 50 to 69. After age 69, however, mammography screening offers minimal gains in life expectancy, and there are potential harms associated with screening that might outweigh the potential benefits. But what should the woman between the ages of 40 and 49 do? For this cohort, evidence that mammography reduces mortality from breast cancer is weak, and the absolute benefit of screening is smaller than it is for the older woman. Proponents and critics adhering to their position continue to enrich the debate. But it is important to understand that they are basing their recommendations on population-based statistics derived from openly acknowledged studies with inherent methodological flaws, and strikingly different conclusions about the benefits of mammography screening for women in their 40s have emerged from the debate. (See a listing of guidelines at the end of this chapter for more information on this issue.)

Breast Cancer Screening Guidelines for the Older Woman

Almost half of new cases and nearly two-thirds of deaths from breast cancer occur in women older than age 50. While the overwhelming majority of breast cancer recommendations agree that mammogram screening is beneficial among women aged 50 and older, after what age is a mammogram screening not worthwhile? The 70-plus age cohort presents a different set of issues. Women in their 70s are different from those in their 60s. Due to differences in health status (e.g., different chronic conditions such as hypertension, cardiac diseases, diabetes) and overall life expectancy among women in this age cohort, the margin of benefit from screening mammography varies widely.[9,10] The life expectancy benefit of screening mammography among women aged 70 to 79 is 40 to 72% of that among women aged 50 to 69.[11] That being said, healthy older women with favorable life expectancies may indeed benefit from continued screening mammography unlike those with substantial chronic diseases.[12]

We do know that breast cancer incidence decreases after age 75.[13] We also know that there are reports of higher rates of overdiagnosis of both invasive breast cancer and DCIS among women aged 60 and older compared to younger women.[14] Given the likelihood that women over age 70 have multiple chronic diseases that could affect survival, it is far more likely that death from causes other than breast cancer would occur. With reduced life expectancy at this age, in all probability screening for breast cancer would not likely affect overall mortality.

Although the data are limited, it is generally agreed that mammograms after age 69 offer little benefit in terms of gains in life expectancy. Based on this thinking, and prior to 2020, several organizations set recommendations for screening older women. Given the uncertainty determining the value of mammography among the older woman, it may not be surprising that professional guidelines vary in their recommendations about setting upper age limits for screening. The American Cancer Society (ACS) recommends stopping screening when life expectancy is less than 10 years. How one accurately determines this is another question that the ACS did not answer! The U.S. Preventive Services Task Force (USPSTF) has determined that there is insufficient evidence to recommend for or against screening women 75 years and older, and most European screening programs stop inviting women for screening between ages 69 and 74 years.

In early 2020, a large-scale, population-based observational study based on over one million Medicare beneficiaries aged 70 to 84 years was published.[15] The researchers found a benefit in screening women aged 70 to 74 years, but not in screening women aged 75 to 84 years. That is, screening past age 75 does not result in substantial reductions in breast cancer mortality compared with stopping screening. One caveat needs to be mentioned so as not to present misleading information. The data from which the analysis was done are based on 1999 to 2008 information. This is important to note because during this time period digital mammography was being introduced. Most mammography done today is digital, which improves the ability to detect cancer and has a lower false positive rate compared to conventional mammography.

From a purely economic point of view, the central question is whether extending mammography screening beyond and into the 70s represents a value. Of course it depends on "value" to whom. Clearly, the choices women in their late 60s and 70s make will vary depending on how each assesses the potential benefits and potential harms of continuing to be screened. This is a personal choice that should be made in consultation with one's physician. Speaking personally, given that my mother died of breast cancer, I am very comfortable having an annual mammogram done into my 70s even though I understand that it may not be necessary to do so. It's personal for me, and each older woman will have to make that decision when the time comes.

Breast Screening Guidelines for Women in Different Racial/Ethnic Groups

The literature is clear that women in low socioeconomic groups, those who do not have health insurance, and those who are from ethnic minorities have comparatively higher rates of breast cancer and higher death rates from breast cancer and are less likely to have a mammogram than white women. Key findings from multiple studies looking at ethnic/racial differences in breast cancer rates show that overall Asian Pacific women have the lowest incidence and death rate from breast cancer compared to women of other racial/ethnic groups; however, within the Asian ethnicities, there is marked variability in the demographics and clinico-pathological features of breast cancer. Asian Pacific combines numerous Asian ethnicities into one group. The determination of race/ethnicity can be problematic, arbitrary, and subject to error and can mask differences within ethnic groupings. In fact, breast cancer-specific mortality among Asian American women has been shown to vary according to Asian ethnicity and breast cancer subtype.[16] That being said, breast cancer incidence and mortality are much lower among this ethnic group compared to others.

Disparities among African American and white women in the United States have long been noted. Breast cancer incidence rates are higher among African American women than among white women and Hispanic women (as was the case with the Asian Pacific category, the Hispanic group combines many different ethnicities into one group, which masks differences among various ethnicities). The breast cancer incidence rate before age 45 is higher among African American women than among white women, whereas between the ages of 60 and 84, the breast cancer incidence rate is much higher in white women than in African American women.[17] The median age of diagnosis for African American women is 59 compared to 63 for white women. Overall, the incidence and death rates for breast cancer are comparatively lower among women of other racial/ethnic groups compared to African American women.

Regarding detection among African American and white women, breast cancer was more likely to be found at an earlier stage among white women than among African American women. This could possibly be due to the fact that white women are more likely to have a mammogram at any age compared to African American women. In terms of type of breast cancer, African American women are more likely than white women to get triple-negative breast cancer, a type of breast cancer that is aggressive and has a poor survival rate.[18] Within the United States, breast cancer rates are higher in African American women than in white women in every state, but especially in seven states: Alabama, Kentucky, Louisiana, Mississippi, Missouri, Oklahoma, and Tennessee. Possible explanations for this include an increase in estrogen receptor (ER)–positive breast cancers in African American women as well as rising rates of obesity, especially among this cohort.

Although breast cancer mortality has decreased among all major racial/ethnic groups, differences persist. Overall, the ethnic/racial disparity has been relatively constant over the past decade. Among women aged 60 to 69 years old, breast cancer death rates dropped 2% per year among white women, compared with 1% per year among African American women. However, the African American-white disparity in breast cancer death rates has increased over time; by 2012, death rates were 42% higher in African American women than in white women.[19]

Hispanic women have about a 20% lower incidence of breast cancer than the general population of the United States.[20] Despite the low incidence compared to the national average, breast cancer is still the most common cancer among Hispanic women, and they share similar risk factors for developing breast cancer with African American women, even though they have a lower incidence rate. Regarding mortality, even though breast cancer is the leading cause of death among Hispanic women, the rate is 25 to 30% lower compared to the U.S. population.

The African American–white women breast cancer disparity is probably a result of a complex interaction of biologic and non-biologic factors, including differences in breast cancer tumor types, stage at diagnosis, obesity, and comorbidity. Among some women, lack of knowledge of breast cancer and breast cancer screening is a barrier, as is lack of health insurance. Certainly, access to and availability of mammogram screening, insurance status, and knowledge of the importance of screening are other factors that to some degree impact the disparities. Poverty, too, is a contributor to breast cancer mortality and is an important factor driving health disparities, and minority women are more likely to live in poverty than white women.

Who Is More Likely to Have a Mammogram?

While the debate about when breast screening should begin and how frequently it should be performed continues, it is interesting to take a look at who actually gets screened. In one of the most detailed and largest studies to quantify the extent to which women follow breast screening recommendations, researchers from the Harvard Medical School found that only 6% of women who received a mammogram in 1992 continued to have regular mammograms over the ensuing 10 years.[21] This finding was based on over 72,000 women of all ages who received screening mammography at the Massachusetts General Hospital between 1985 and 2002. Only 1 in 20 women consistently followed the recommendations for annual mammography.

The study also found that among those women diagnosed with invasive breast cancer, those who had annual mammograms had a lower risk of death (approximately 12%) compared to those who received mammograms every 2 years (approximately 16%) or every 5 years (approximately 25%). It should be said that this cohort would not necessarily be generalizable to the general population. These women were diagnosed with cancer and had much more motivation and reason to continue with screening. Further, the study was conducted almost 20 years ago, and probably things have changed since then.

In the past, African American women were less likely than white women to get regular mammograms, and lower screening rates in the past could be a possible reason for the difference in survival rates today. However, recent data from the Centers for Disease Control and Prevention (CDC) show marked improvement in mammogram screening among all racial/ethnic groups. The "good" news is that as of 2015, two-thirds of all women aged 40 and over had a mammogram within the past two years.[22] Approximately, 65% of white women, 70% of African American women, and 61% of Hispanic women over age 40 had a mammogram within the past two years, indicating no substantial difference among the racial/ethnic groups. However, even after accounting for factors that could explain differences in survival (i.e., past screening rates, access to care), African American women continue to be diagnosed with more advanced breast cancers and have worse survival than white American women.[23] Among Hispanic women, rates of breast cancer and breast cancer mortality are lower compared to Black/non-Hispanic Black and white/non-Hispanic white women.[24] However, breast cancer is still the most common cancer (and the leading cause of cancer death) among Hispanic/Latina women, so screening is just as important for Latina women as it is for African American and white women.

Breast Cancer and Breast Screening among Lesbian, Gay, and Bisexual Women

Lesbian, gay, and bisexual (LGB) women might be at greater risk for breast cancer not because of their sexual orientation, but because they have certain risk factors (i.e., never having children or having children later in life) that would put them at higher risk of developing breast cancer. Counseling LGB women about breast cancer and breast cancer screening is important, especially since some individuals might think that because they are gay or bisexual they do not necessarily need to be screened. They do need to be screened. Regardless of their sexual orientation, they are female, which puts them at a potential risk of developing breast cancer. And African American LGB women are especially at risk, making it even more important that they get regular screening.

To a large extent, we do not have good data to show breast cancer incidence among LGB. The large national cancer registries and surveys do not collect data about sexual orientation. Complicating things, there are many factors that might discourage LGB women from getting screened. Some individuals may be embarrassed to go for screening; some may feel (rightly or wrongly) that in the past they have been treated insensitively by physicians and other health personnel. Some may feel that because they are gay or bisexual they have been victims of discrimination by the medical profession. The medical profession needs to understand better LGB concerns and to stress the importance of early detection without judgment or stigma.

Some studies show that mammography screening rates among LGB and heterosexual women are similar: 79% of LGB women aged 50 to 74 had a mammogram in the past 2 years compared to 73% of straight women aged 50 to 74.[25] However, the evidence is scant since most databases do not have information about sexual orientation, making it difficult to ascertain the extent to which LGB women get regular mammograms.

There are websites that address the needs and concerns of LGB women regarding breast cancer and breast cancer screening (i.e., Living beyond Breast Cancer; https://www.lbbc.org/i-am-lgbt-breast-cancer), and the National LGBT Cancer Network has helpful information about cancer and the LGBT community (https://cancer-network.org/cancer-information/cancer-resources-for-the-lgbt-community/). There is not enough information available about transgender individuals and breast cancer, which is why it is not discussed here.

Breast Cancer Screening among Women with Physical Disabilities

Women with physical disabilities tend to get mammograms less often than women without such limitations perhaps because of lack of access to mammography centers that meet their needs.[26] Women living with a disability, compared to women without disabilities, may face challenges that make it hard to get a mammogram, including how to manage if she uses a wheelchair or a scooter or is unable to stand and must be screened while seated. In an effort to assist women with disabilities, the CDC prepared a tip sheet to provide information about mammogram screening for those with physical disabilities.[27]

Barriers to Screening That Women Face

In order for women, regardless of age and ethnic group, to be an informed and active participant in the decision-making process to get screened, they need to understand the range of uncertainties for both the potential benefits and the potential harms of mammography. An international survey of women living in the United States, the United Kingdom, Italy, and Switzerland found that a high proportion of women overestimated the benefits of screening.[28] Most of the women seemed to be poorly informed about the potential benefits of screening.[29] Common misconceptions about mammography include: screening tests are meant for patients with known symptoms; screening reduces the incidence of breast cancer; early detection implies reduced mortality; all breast cancers progress; screening tests are for women with symptoms; screening reduces the incidence of breast cancer; and mammograms can cause cancer.

What barriers (perceived and actual) prevent women from getting screened? What barriers are similar across racial/ethnic groups, and which barriers differ among the groups? There have been many studies conducted to identify factors that serve to keep women from getting screened. The reasons for not getting a mammogram are not necessarily specific to one racial/ethnic group or sexual orientation.

A large-scale review of published studies identified 19 plausible factors that serve as barriers to mammography, which were then categorized into three groups: personal attitudes and beliefs, accessibility and associated factors, and social influence.[30] Personal attitudes and beliefs included fear of getting a positive mammogram result. Accessibility and associated factors included factors such as the cost of the mammogram, availability, and transportation. Social influence included lack of physician recommendation for a mammogram and cultural beliefs. Another study, published after eight years, later took into account barriers across race/ethnicity.[31] The researchers categorized barriers into four groups: psychological/knowledge related, logistical, cultural/immigration related, and social/interpersonal. In this scheme, the psychological/knowledge-related barrier is similar to the previously categorized personal attitudes and beliefs category, and the logistical barrier is similar to the accessibility and associated factors group. The social influence barrier was expanded to include cultural factors.

Findings found that overall, fear was a common barrier expressed by women in all racial/ethnic groups, as was procrastination. Lack of knowledge/misinformation about mammography screening was reported more frequently by African American and Hispanic women. Of the logistical barriers, cost and lack of insurance were most frequently reported by all women in all racial/ethnic groups.

African American women most often reported psychological/knowledge-related barriers such as fear of getting a mammogram, fear of pain/discomfort/embarrassment of the procedure, and financial issues that precluded them from getting screened. Among Hispanic women, lack of knowledge was a primary barrier as was cost of the procedure. Women in these racial/ethnic groups also reported negative/rude attitudes from the providers; women reported that white women were treated better.

In order to improve perceptions about mammography and to encourage women, particularly minority women, to get screened, the above factors must be considered in order to remove the perceived barriers to mammography. Tailoring messages that are culturally relevant also would be an important step in improving acceptance of breast screening.

What Does This All Mean?

The question of who should be screened for breast cancer, at what age, and how often is not simply an academic debate. There are factors other than the statistical results of a trial that must be taken into account. We know that there are differences among racial/ethnic groups, which need to be addressed. Given that minority women, especially African American women, have poorer prognosis primarily because their breast cancers are detected at a later stage and that they tend to have more aggressive types of breast cancer, perhaps screening for these women should be done while they are in their 40s. We know that LGB women present with different needs and have different concerns about mammogram screening, and women with physical disabilities have unique issues that need to be addressed so as to enable them to get screened.

Part of the problem is that women receive inaccurate or conflicting messages about the benefits of screening. If the experts cannot agree on the value of mammography, what is the layperson expected to understand? When one set of recommendations says women should get screened annually from age 45 on, and another set of recommendations says screening should not start until age 50, the mixed messages only serve to confuse and maybe even scare the layperson. Also, the issue of false positive and false negative results is glossed over, and there is little information about possible adverse effects of screening.[32] One study that looked at the information presented on the Internet by major breast cancer advocacy groups and consumer organizations found that most were "informational poor" and severely biased in favor of screening.[33] An honest and clear explanation of the potential benefits and potential harms is needed before informed decisions can be made about whether to get screened, at what age, and how often?

What Does This Mean for Me?

As the following will show, there is no uniformity in screening guidelines among organizations that have published guidelines, although all strongly endorse the value of mammography screening. Key questions, which remain under debate, include: At what age should a woman be screened? How frequently should a woman be screened? The evidence from the large trials, flaws and all, can be interpreted to support screening beginning at age 40 or age 45 or age 50. Yet, there is no agreement regarding the "best" age to begin screening. The truth is that "one size does not fit all."

Mammography's benefits must be weighed against the potential harms (clinical, financial, and emotional). We know that African American women are at higher risk for developing a particularly aggressive form of breast cancer at a young age. Should consideration should be given to adjusting breast cancer screening guidelines to reflect this? None of the screening recommendations take into account age-specific patterns based on race/ethnicity. Should consideration be given to adjusting breast cancer screening guidelines based not just on age, but also race/ethnicity?[34]

While we now have so much knowledge about the potential benefits (and, yes, harms) of mammography, there are still so many unanswered questions. In terms of treatment for breast cancer, tremendous advances have been made over the last decade or so, which should be encouraging and good news to those with breast cancer. Subsequent chapters will explore these issues.

Current Breast Cancer Screening Guidelines

Several organizations have published breast cancer screening guidelines, albeit with some differences in recommendations.

- **American Cancer Society (ACS) Breast Cancer Guidelines, 2019**

    (See https://www.cancer.org/latest-news/special-coverage /american-cancer-society-breast-cancer-screening-guidelines .html.)

    In 2015, the ACS made changes to their breast cancer screening guideline by recommending that women **at average risk** for breast cancer start annual screening with mammograms at age 45, instead of age 40 (which was the starting age in their previous guideline). The change was made based on evidence showing that the risk of cancer is lower for women aged 40 to 44 and the risk of harm from screenings (biopsies for false positive findings, overdiagnosis) is somewhat higher. Because of this, the ACS made the recommendation that screening beginning at age 40 was no longer warranted. That being said, the ACS states that women between the ages of 40 to 44 can choose to begin getting mammograms yearly if they want to. Overall, the ACS concluded that the balance of benefits to risks becomes more favorable at age 45, which is why they recommend that annual screening begin at this age.

    Women ages 40 to 44 should have the choice to start annual breast cancer screening with mammograms (x-rays of the breast) *if they wish to do so* [italics added].
    Women age 45 to 54 should get mammograms every year.

Women 55 and older should switch to mammograms every 2 years, or can continue yearly screening. Screening should continue as long as a woman is in good health and is expected to live 10 more years or longer.

Since most women are postmenopausal by age 55 and because the evidence does not show a statistical advantage to annual screening in postmenopausal women, the ACS guidelines committee concluded that women should move to screening every two years starting at age 55. That being said, the guideline makes clear that women may choose to continue screening every year after age 55 if they so choose.

The ACS issued separate guidelines for women who are *at high risk* for breast cancer, including having *BRCA1* or *BRCA2* gene mutation based on having had genetic testing; have a first-degree relative (parent, brother, sister, or child) with a *BRCA1* or *BRCA2* gene mutation and not have had genetic testing themselves; had radiation therapy to the chest when they were between the ages of 10 and 30 years; have Li-Fraumeni syndrome, Cowden syndrome, or Bannayan-Riley-Ruvalcaba syndrome; or have first-degree relatives with one of these syndromes. Women with these risk factors should get a breast MRI and a mammogram every year, typically starting at age 30. If MRI is used, it should be in addition to, not instead of, a screening mammogram. This is because although an MRI is more likely to detect cancer than a mammogram, it may still miss some cancers that a mammogram would detect. The ACS recommends against MRI screening for women whose lifetime risk of breast cancer is less than 15%.

- **The U.S. Preventive Services Task Force Final Recommendation for Breast Cancer Screening (USPSTF)**

    (See https://www.uspreventiveservicestaskforce.org/Page /Document/RecommendationStatementFinal/breast-cancer -screening1.)

    The USPSTF is the leading independent panel of private sector experts in prevention and primary care. It conducts rigorous and impartial assessments of scientific evidence for a broad range of preventive services. The USPSTF updated its breast cancer screening recommendations in 2019, recommending biennial screening mammography for women aged 50 to 74 years. The Task Force's screening recommendation for women younger than age 50 years stipulates that this decision should be an individual one. The rationale for this decision rests on the belief that while screening mammography in women aged 40 to 49 years may reduce the risk for breast cancer death, the number of deaths averted is smaller than that in older women and the number of false positive results and unnecessary biopsies is larger. The balance of benefits and harms is likely to improve as women move from their early to late 40s. Regarding screening for women 75 years and older, the USP-STF concluded that the current evidence is insufficient to assess the balance of benefits and harms of screening mammography in older women. The USPSTF makes it clear in the body of its recommendations that clinical decisions involve more considerations than evidence alone. While clinicians should understand the evidence of clinical benefits and harms, they should individualize decision-making to the specific patient or situation.

- **The American College of Physicians (ACP) Screening for Breast Cancer in Average-Risk Women: A Guidance Statement**

  The ACP, the national professional organization of internists, critically reviewed the evidence on breast cancer screening so as to assist clinicians in making decisions about breast cancer screening in asymptomatic women with average risk for breast cancer.[35] Four guidelines were issued:

  > *Guidance Statement 1:* In average-risk women aged 40 to 49 years, clinicians should discuss whether to screen for breast cancer with mammography before age 50 years. Discussion should include the potential benefits and harms and a woman's preferences. The potential harms outweigh the benefits in most women aged 40 to 49 years.
  > *Guidance Statement 2:* In average-risk women aged 50 to 74 years, clinicians should offer screening for breast cancer with biennial mammography.
  > *Guidance Statement 3:* In average-risk women aged 75 years or older or in women with a life expectancy of 10 years or less, clinicians should discontinue screening for breast cancer.
  > *Guidance Statement 4:* In average-risk women of all ages, clinicians should not use clinical breast examination to screen for breast cancer.

- **The American Society of Breast Surgeons Issues Updated Breast Cancer Screening Guidelines**

  (See https://www.breastsurgeons.org/docs/statements/Position-Statement-on-Screening-Mammography.pdf.)

  The American Society of Breast Surgeons issued breast cancer screening guidelines at their annual meeting in May 2019. Their recommendations are that women older than age 25 should undergo formal risk assessment for breast cancer (not clearly specified); that women with an average risk of breast cancer should begin yearly screening at age 40; that women with a higher-than-average risk of breast cancer should begin yearly screening with mammography and be offered yearly supplemental imaging and that this screening should be initiated at a risk-based age (not clearly specified); and that screening mammography should cease when life expectancy is <10 years.

- **The American College of Radiology (ACR) and the Society of Breast Imaging (SBI) Guidelines**

  The ACR and the SBI issued detailed recommendations for breast cancer screening for women at average risk of breast cancer and for women at high risk of developing breast cancer.[36] For average-risk women, the ACR and SBI recommend an annual mammogram beginning at age 40, and for women at increased risk, yearly mammograms starting by age 30 (but not before age 25). Ultrasound and MRI in addition to mammography can be considered in high-risk women.

CHAPTER SEVEN

To Screen or Not to Screen: Changing Advice on Mammography Screening

Although the previous chapters presented information on the various modalities that are being used to detect breast cancer, it is mammography (flat screen and digital) that remains the most widespread technique for population-based screening. The other modalities may at some point replace mammography, but at this moment in time, most of the other options should only be used for women who are at high risk for developing breast cancer. For women with minimal risk of developing breast cancer, those modalities would be overkill, and they are much more costly than mammography.

Each woman is unique, and her risk of breast cancer will vary by many factors, including age, family history, genetics, and biology. For example, the annual risk of a 60-year old woman being diagnosed with breast cancer is greater than that of a 45-year old, and the older woman has a greater likelihood of dying from the disease. Mammogram screening recommendations logically need to reflect these differences. But there is an ongoing debate among breast cancer researchers and clinicians about the "value" of mammography. The issue of optimal intervals between screening mammograms is not uniformly agreed upon by physicians and cancer organizations such as the American Cancer Society, and this can send mixed messages to the public. Who should be screened? At what age? How frequently?

The Mammography Dilemma

The long-term effectiveness of mammogram screening and its effect on survival in particular are subject to differences of opinion despite the fact that these opinions are based on the same data sets. Rational decision-making, be it for the individual or for population groups, should be based on sound data, but if there are disagreements in interpretation of the data, things get much more complicated. If the data on which policy recommendations are made are suspect or flawed, decision-making will naturally be compromised. This issue is central to the mammogram controversy. If the experts cannot agree, what is the layperson supposed to believe?

As was stated many times in previous chapters, an assessment of the potential benefits of screening and the potential harms needs to be taken into account. Clearly, if the harms outweigh the benefits, screening should not be offered. If early detection does not result in better outcomes, there would be no point in offering screening. If there is evidence that screening results in better outcomes but only for a small number of individuals, the harms of screening on a widespread scale need to be assessed. With mammography screening, there is a potentially large benefit for a small number of individuals and a potentially small amount of harm for a much larger number. Because screening involves primarily healthy women, the potential benefits and harms must be taken into account, and the limitations of the screening technology should be acknowledged.

The benefit of mammogram screening focuses on detecting breast cancer at an early stage so that treatment can begin with the hope and expectation of extending lives. Increased survival is the basic premise of early disease detection. While screening for any disease does not necessarily reduce the risk for being diagnosed with the disease, it is meant to reduce the risk for dying of the disease. Does mammography do this? It depends on who you ask!

There have been numerous studies and clinical trials that have compared breast cancer mortality among women who were screened to those who were not. There have been hundreds of opinion pieces and editorials commenting on the findings of these studies. Yes, the trials differed in many ways, including how women were randomized and how the data were analyzed; however, there is general agreement, albeit not uniform agreement, that screening mammography for women aged 50 to 69 is beneficial. That is, the benefits of screening outweigh the harms of not screening. There are differences of opinion, however, regarding recommendations for women younger than age 50. And there have been some experts who have questioned the value of mammography screening for women of any age. Yes, there is a lot of confusion and disagreement.

Consider a woman in her mid-40s with an average risk of breast cancer. Should she have annual mammogram screenings? Would the benefits of mammography justify the potential harms, such as a false positive test result that would trigger additional testing? Certainly detecting breast cancer at an early stage is important and potentially beneficial, but this woman has no way of knowing whether in the next decade she will be one of the majority who does not develop breast cancer or one of the few who will. The data, which will be discussed in more detail later on, seem to indicate that regular screening confers only a small benefit for the average woman in her 40s who is not considered to be at high risk for developing breast cancer in her lifetime. But what may be a marginal benefit epidemiologically speaking may not be perceived as such by the individual. Her concerns and her needs are much more personal than the impersonal, dispassionate nature of probability that epidemiology relies on.

In order to understand the crux of the dilemma, it is important to know what the large clinical trials have concluded. These randomized clinical trials rely on comparing a similar group of subjects, one group of which will be randomized to receive the treatment (e.g., mammography screening) and the other group to serve as a control. Hundreds of thousands of women from many different countries have participated in screening trials since the early 1960s.

The Health Insurance Plan of New York (HIP) randomized clinical trial was the first to examine the feasibility of mammography as a population-based screening tool. HIP was a prepaid group insurance entity, which means that individuals had their medical bills covered by HIP and care delivered by HIP doctors. As such, there was a defined population whose medical records and insurance claims were in the HIP system. This rich database enabled researchers to obtain necessary data easily and longitudinally follow participants over time. The database was perfect for a randomized trial because the target population was easily identified.

The HIP trial, the first large-scale population-based randomized clinical mammography trial, was conducted between 1963 and 1967 at a time when routine mammography was not offered.[1] Physicians would order a mammogram to help with the diagnosis of possible breast cancer. A positive mammogram would then result in a surgeon performing a biopsy. Essentially, the mammogram served as a diagnostic tool, not a screening tool. In the HIP study, approximately 60,000 to 62,000 women (the actual number of women in the trial is unclear, as it has been reported differently in publications) aged 40 to 64 were matched on key variables and randomized into one of two groups: the intervention group received an annual clinical breast exam and screening mammography over the course of 4 years. The control group received usual care. The follow-up period was as long as 18 years, which is sufficient time for breast cancer to develop in this cohort of women.

The major findings from this trial served to validate the benefits of population-based mammography screening.[2] Specifically, findings showed that those women who were randomized to the mammography group had more early-stage breast cancers detected compared to women who were in the control group: 70% of the screened women with localized breast cancer compared to 45% in the control group. The most important finding, however, was that the death rate from breast cancer among those who had mammogram screening was between 30 and 40% lower than that for those in the control group.[3] That is, of the approximately 31,000 women who were not screened, 124 died of breast cancer compared with 81 of the approximately 31,000 who were screened. While these numbers may not appear on surface to be substantial, statistically they are. The study showed statistically that screening asymptomatic women for breast cancer could cut the breast cancer death rate significantly.

No study is perfect, and the HIP study certainly had its limitations. Although randomization should have produced equal distribution of women in the two groups, there were significant imbalances in the distribution of women with prior breast lumps, age at menopause, and education. Ideally, the groups should have been very similar in important variables at baseline, but they were not. Furthermore, researchers decided that they did not want to include women who already had breast cancer, and these women were dropped from the study after they were randomized. About 1,100 women were dropped—800 from the mammography group and 300 from the control group. Hence, more women with preexisting breast cancer were excluded from the screening group than from the control group, which could introduce bias in favor of the screening group and affect the findings.

Moreover, when the data were examined more closely, it became apparent that the decreased death rate occurred more frequently among women aged 50 and older. There was no statistically significant difference in mortality among those in their 40s. Hence, there was a dilemma: given that there was no difference in mortality among those younger than age 50, should mammography be encouraged for this age cohort? There were those who concluded that the HIP study did not support the use of screening mammography in women aged 40 to 50.[4] Clearly, more studies are needed to be done to help clarify this issue.

In 1972, a year after the landmark HIP study was published, and after President Richard Nixon signed into law the Cancer Control Act, the American Cancer Society (ACS) and National Cancer Institute (NCI) joined forces to implement another large-scale breast cancer screening study. The Breast Cancer Detection Demonstration Project (BCDDP), a national mammography screening project that ran from 1973 to 1981 in 29 centers across the United States, was designed to screen over a quarter of a million American women.[5] This massive study aimed to provide evidence on mammography's impact on breast cancer mortality among women in different age groups. The ACS took the lead on designing the study and made the decision to include women as young as age 35. Rather than conducting a randomized controlled trial, as was done in the HIP study, the ACS chose to conduct a demonstration project to assess the feasibility of periodic screening of large numbers of women for breast cancer. Efforts were made to include poor and minority women in this study, a cohort that was underrepresented in the HIP study. Women were screened annually for five years.

Findings showed that mammography was very effective in identifying most cancers in all age groups, but it was more effective in so doing among older women (age 50 and older). High survival rates were observed among the 4,240 women with histologically confirmed diagnosis of breast cancer, indicating that the cancer was found at an early, treatable stage. The relative 5-, 8-, and 10-year survival rates were 88%, 83%, and 79%, respectively. It seems that there were substantial gains in survival primarily because a high proportion of cancers were being diagnosed and treated at an early stage.

The study looked carefully at the value of screening women before age 50 and compared breast cancers that were detected as well as survival rates between those women younger than age 50 to those in their 50s and older. Data showed that screening was as effective in the younger woman as in the older woman. However, mammography did not detect 10% of cancers in women younger than age 50 compared to 5% in women older than age 50.[6] Despite its flaws, this project was hailed as a huge success, with the media proclaiming that breast cancer screening is saving lives.

While more studies were needed to validate the benefits of mammography among asymptomatic women, two major events in the mid-1970s probably did more to encourage women to have a mammogram than anything else. Within a few years of each other, both Betty Ford and Happy Rockefeller were diagnosed with breast cancer, and both had a mastectomy. The tremendous publicity of these events served to galvanize women to have a mammogram. While the early breast cancer screening studies served to affirm the benefits of regular mammogram screening, it was the personal experience of Mrs. Ford and Mrs. Rockefeller and their willingness to talk about their breast cancer experience that provided the impetus for women to be screened.

While the benefits of mammogram were being touted, there were skeptics who made their concerns and criticisms known. Dr. John C. Bailar III, a physician who also had credentials in biostatistics and epidemiology, was the NCI's deputy associate director for cancer control at the time. He published a piece questioning the HIP findings, writing that the study had not definitively determined the benefits of screening mammography.[7] From a statistical perspective, he felt that the value of the screening test was exaggerated because many slow-growing lesions were unlikely to ever become clinically significant breast cancers (this relates to issues of lead time and length bias that was discussed in a previous chapter). He also challenged the findings of the BCDDP, citing that the methodology was flawed (i.e., issues with study design and study population). The BCDDP was not a randomized clinical trial, rather an uncontrolled demonstration project with biases inherent in such a study. Bailar argued that data from this uncontrolled study would not permit meaningful conclusions.

Others, even those at the NCI, also questioned the benefit of routine mammographic screening in women under age 50, based on findings from the HIP study and the BCDDP project.[8] In response, the ACS and NCI decided to offer mammography only to those under age 50 who were "at high risk." How one defined "high risk" also was a point of contention.

While the debate continued in the United States, four randomized trials were initiated in Europe and Canada from 1977 to 1983 with the purpose of investigating the potential benefits of mammography screening. The Malmö Mammographic Screening Trial (MMST) in Sweden began in 1976 and lasted 12 years.[9] Approximately 21,000 women were randomized to the screening group and 21,200 to the control group. The randomization produced similar groups. Women with preexisting breast cancer were excluded from the screening group, but not from the control group. A second Swedish trial, the Stockholm trial begun in 1981, focused on women aged 40 to 64.[10] Women with preexisting breast cancer were excluded from the screened group but not from the control group. Randomization was based on date of birth, with women born on days 11 through 20 of any month comprising the control group. There was substantial discrepancy of the actual number of women in each group, and the number of women in the screened group declined by 2,000 individuals and rose by 1,000 individuals in the control group over the course of the trial. The researchers could not explain this inconsistency, but it certainly appears that the randomization method was flawed.

A third Swedish trial, the Gothenburg trial, begun in 1982, followed women between the ages of 40 and 49 for 11 years.[11] Despite randomization, women in the screened group were significantly younger than those in the control group. Women with preexisting breast cancer were excluded from the screened group but not from the control group. Findings showed that women in the control group had a higher cancer incidence than the screened group, and there were higher than expected cancer incidence in both groups. There are two other trials conducted in Kopparberg and Ostergotland, which will not be discussed here because there were methodological flaws inherent in these studies.

Overall, between 1976 and 1982 four randomized mammography screening trials at five screening centers (Malmo, Kopparberg, Ostergotland, Stockholm, and Gothenburg) started in Sweden with the aim of determining whether screening could reduce breast cancer mortality. All four trials had a similar design, using mammography alone as the primary screening tool. Overall, findings showed a statistically significant reduction in breast cancer mortality among women who received screening, but there were methodological flaws inherent in each of the trials, which to some degree compromises the findings.[12]

The Edinburgh trial started in 1976 and followed women between the ages of 45 and 64 for up to 10 years.[13,14] Approximately 23,200 women were in the screened group and 21,900 in the control group. Cluster randomization was based on physician practices. Criticism of this trial focused on the method of randomization, especially since the groups differed substantially at baseline. This is considered by epidemiologists and statisticians to be a fatal flaw—groups must be similar after randomization; otherwise, it is difficult to accept the study findings. It would be like comparing apples to oranges. Additionally, there were socioeconomic differences between study and control groups, as only 26% of the women in the control group were in the highest socioeconomic group, whereas 53% of those in the screened group were in the highest socioeconomic group. And there were more women with preexisting breast cancer who were excluded from the screened group than from the control group. Because of these factors, this trial is considered to be highly flawed and the findings suspect.

The first Canadian National Breast Screening study began in 1980. This trial at the time was the only one to specifically study women aged 40 to 49 and to evaluate the efficacy of annual mammography, breast physical exam, and instruction of breast self-exam in reducing breast cancer mortality.[15] That is, breast cancer mortality would be compared between (1) women who received screening with annual mammography and breast self-exam and (2) women who received community care after a single breast exam by a physician and instruction on breast self-exam. Of the 50,430 women who volunteered to be in the study, approximately 25,000 were randomized to the screening group and 25,000 to the control group (usual care with annual follow-up). Before randomization, each woman received an initial breast exam by a physician and instruction on how to do a breast self-exam. The groups were similar at baseline.

Women were followed for up to 16 years. Those who had a mammogram did not have reduced breast cancer mortality compared to those who did not have a mammogram. This was a dramatic finding and was the first to show limited benefit of mammography. The researchers concluded that based on the findings, there was no statistical benefit of mammography in women under age 50.

The second Canadian National Breast Screening study, which started in 1980, focused on women aged 50 to 59.[16] In this trial, 39,405 women were randomly assigned to receive a mammogram plus breast exam by a physician or a physician clinical exam only. The groups were evenly matched (approximately 20,000 randomized to each group), and the average follow-up was 13 years (ranging from 11 to 16 years). This study also showed that mammography had apparently no impact on breast cancer mortality. The Canadian studies were the only ones to show no benefit in mortality reduction, a fact that had to be tested further in other studies.

In summary, each of the preceding large trials used different methodologies, to some degree had methodological flaws that one could argue compromised the findings, and focused on somewhat different cohorts of women. Not surprisingly, perhaps, the trials did not help quell the debate about mammography's worth. Opinions were not changed. Physicians and surgeons who treated breast cancer patients strongly advocated for mammography, probably because they saw firsthand women who died of the disease. They believed that mammography was beneficial. However, others argued that just because a mammogram detected a lesion, such cancers might never have progressed or progressed to the point that the woman would die of breast cancer.

Trying to resolve the debate about the value of mammography, the National Institutes of Health (NIH) organized a consensus conference in 1977. A series of such conferences were held in the United States to discuss the issues in an effort to reach a consensus about mammography as a screening tool and whether it causes more harm than good. A consensus panel chaired by Dr. Samuel Thier of Yale University agreed that annual mammographic screening of women over age 50 was appropriate, but women aged 40 to 49 should receive testing only if they had previous breast cancer or had a strong family history of breast cancer. Women aged 35 to 39 should receive mammograms only if they had had breast cancer.[17]

The ACS, American College of Radiology, and other interested organizations continued to recommend annual mammography for women aged 50 to 69. But in 1980, the ACS differed with the NCI and went on record to advocate that women aged 35 to 39 should get a baseline mammogram and that women aged 40 to 49 have a mammogram every one to two years. Even though the findings from various studies were not conclusive, primarily a result of flaws in the methodology used, the ACS nevertheless went on record to state that mammography can save lives in both older and younger women. It was apparent at the time that there was a serious difference in opinion about mammography screening's value, especially in women younger than age 50. The consensus panels did not produce uniformity in recommendations after all.

In 1988, the NCI, the American College of Radiology, and 11 other medical organizations went on record to recommend routine screening mammograms for younger women. However in the early 1990s, a meta-analysis that included data from the eight trials that had been published (e.g., pooling the results of each into one analysis) led to the conclusion that mammography did not show a benefit, particularly for women younger than age 50.[18] Based on this study, the NCI changed its mind and withdrew its support for routine mammograms for women under age 50.

The meta-analysis did not quell the debate, and it got nasty, with some calling the NCI's decision a death sentence for women. The proponents of mammography argued that screening women in their 40s reduced deaths from breast cancer. While opponents of mammography did not necessarily refute this, they argued that 2,500 healthy women under age 50 would have to receive regular screening in order to extend one's life and it would result in many unnecessary tests being done to rule in or rule out cancer.[19] To further complicate things, in 1997, the ACS changed its recommendations and went on record to advise women in their 40s to get a mammogram every year. The American College of Radiology also agreed with this recommendation. But the U.S. Preventive Services Task Force opposed routine screening in younger women in favor of individualized case assessment.

To Screen or Not to Screen: This Is the Big Question

Based on years of following hundreds of thousands of women and accumulating mounds of data, what conclusions can be drawn regarding the effect of mammography screening on breast cancer mortality? One of the basic tenets of screening is improvement in survival. To what extent are lives extended because of early breast cancer mortality? To what extent does mammography screening improve overall survival? Although few of the large-scale trials were methodologically "perfect" (very few studies are "perfect"), most showed varying reductions in breast cancer mortality. Only the Canadian trials failed to find such a benefit, regardless of age of the woman. No differences in survival rates between women who were screened by physical exam compared to women who were screened by physical exam and mammography were found.

The Canadian trials have been heavily criticized perhaps because they were the only ones to show the most negative results. The other large-scale trials generally show that screening is beneficial in that there was a reduction in mortality from breast cancer among women aged 50 and older. What makes the Canadian study findings so different from those from other studies? Why were these trials the only ones to find no beneficial effect from mammography? The findings from Canadian trials were not widely accepted by the medical community nor from most key organizations, including the American Cancer Society. Rather than delve further to try to answer the question, proponents of mammography chose to ignore the Canadian findings and continued to advocate for breast cancer screening for women between the ages of 50 and 69. Recommendations for women younger than age 50 were more controversial.

By 1997, findings from the eight large-scale trials were published, but rather than actually resolving the debate, they served to further muddy the waters. Why do some studies show a benefit and others do not? It could be that the methodological flaws inherent in each study, some more serious than others, contribute to the differences in trial findings. From a methodological perspective, there are certain factors that must be taken into account in order for the study findings to be considered to be meaningful (i.e., statistically valid and reliable). Control of sources of bias must be incorporated into the study design. That is, bias can occur if the selection of the study population is faulty, if the assignment of individuals to treatment or control groups is unequal, or if the method of measuring outcomes or study endpoints is different. For example, the randomization process in most of the trials failed to create similar groups, which is a serious flaw. The actual number of women in each of the groups in some trials could not be determined (i.e., Stockholm, Kopparberg, Ostergotland, and the HIP study), raising questions as to what effect this had on study findings. Differences in training of radiologists and differences in mammography techniques also could be a possible source of bias. It is well known that the skill of the radiologist in reading mammography films varies.

The size of the study population and the duration of the study are important factors. If study findings are based on a small sample of individuals, there will be less statistical relevance and less generalizability. All of the randomized clinical trials included a large number of women, so small sample size is not an issue. Duration of the trial could be an issue, however. Do the trials follow the study population for a long enough period of time for endpoints/outcomes (i.e., death) to occur?

Even though proponents and opponents, all experts in the field, were looking at the same data, they were coming to different conclusions. For some, the problems of the trials raised questions about the reliability of the findings and led them to question the effectiveness of breast cancer screening. A few even advocated that mammograms not be recommended routinely because they do not reduce breast cancer mortality. There was (and continues to be) heated debate about the value of mammography screening among women younger than age 50. Some believe that women in their 40s should receive regular screening and others believe that there was not enough evidence to support routine screening for this cohort, a low-risk population to begin with. Since breast cancer is comparatively rare in this age cohort, any benefit from mammography was likely to be small. However, even though women in their 40s have a lower risk of cancer compared to women older than age 50, the cancers found in the younger women tend to be more aggressive. Would the potential benefit of early mammogram screening be evident among women younger than age 50? The data from the large-scale trials could not answer this question. None of this was helpful to the layperson, especially those younger than age 50, who just wanted to know if she should get screened.

The Crux of the Controversy

In January 2000, Danish researchers at the Nordic Cochrane Center in Copenhagen revisited the issue of breast cancer screening.[20] They critically looked at the individual trials to see if breast cancer mortality had decreased as a result of mammogram screening. It was their opinion that all but two of the trials were so flawed in design that the results of each were unreliable. That is, these studies might have found benefits when in fact there were none, or they might have exaggerated what benefits there were.

The Danish researchers were highly critical of both the randomized methods used in the trials as well as the eligibility criteria used for study population selection. Women, it seems, were more likely to be excluded from the screened group if they had a prior diagnosis of breast cancer. Since any breast cancer survivor has a greater chance of ultimately dying of breast cancer, this could bias the conclusions. Further, in these trials, more women died of causes other than breast cancer than those who died of breast cancer, thus questioning the ability of the trials to detect reliably the impact of mammography on overall mortality. That is, the Danish researchers thought that knowledge of screening status might affect the judgment of cause of death.

The degree to which mammography reduces mortality is an important issue in the mammography debate. Cause of death likely differed among women who were screened compared to those who were not. The Danish researchers concluded that based on their review of the data, screening for breast cancer with mammography did not decrease breast cancer mortality, and therefore screening should not be recommended. This was an explosive conclusion. Screening for breast cancer with mammography was unjustified (their term) because there is no reliable evidence showing that it reduces mortality.

The Danish researchers could find no statistical evidence that screening decreases breast cancer mortality, the main outcome measure in the screening trials. They calculated that for every 1,000 women screened biannually for 12 years, 1 breast cancer death is avoided while the total number of deaths increased by 6. They also criticized the methodological quality of the screening trials, making it difficult to base recommendations on the data.

When the Danish researchers submitted their review to the editors of the Breast Cancer Group of the Cochrane Collaboration based in Oxford, England, the editors insisted on changes that would lend support to the benefits of screening. The Danish researchers refused. The respected journal *The Lancet* did publish the findings as written but also included a review of the Oxford group's concerns.[21] In 2001, the Danish researchers published a reassessment of their findings and again asserted that mammograms do not lead to increased survival. In fact, the researchers concluded that the estimated mammography effect on all-cause mortality was negligible.[22] This second review confirmed and strengthened the previous findings. Of note, the researchers found that women who were screened tended to have more invasive tests done to follow up on inconclusive or suspicious findings from mammogram (i.e., false positive test results). Yet their death rates were no different from those who were not screened. This conclusion directly challenged the traditional belief that mammograms saved lives, which further fueled the debate about the value of mammography.

The Danish critique of the data not only called into question the value of mammography for women younger than age 50; it also threw into doubt the benefit of mammography for older women. Proponents of mammography argued that the flaws inherent in the studies that the Danish researchers discounted were not severe enough to discount the body of evidence, in their opinion. Those who had questioned mammography's value used the Danish findings to bolster their viewpoint, which was that mammography does not improve survival and leads to treatment for tumors that would not have threatened a woman's life if left alone.

The strong anti–mammography screening stance created a furor. All of the recommendations regarding mammogram screening were based on data from the same trials that were included in the Danish reanalysis. As flawed as these studies may be, nonprofit organizations and government agencies involved in setting screening recommendations continued to argue that the benefits of screening far outweighed the negatives. Furthermore, the issue is an emotionally charged one. Saying that mammogram screening does not work goes against deeply held beliefs, especially among women who have been told that mammography saves lives.

Other researchers looking at the contribution of mammography screening to reductions in mortality have concluded that screening does make a difference. Data from the Regional Oncology Centres in Uppsala and Linkoping, Sweden, were used to compare deaths in two Swedish counties from breast cancer diagnosed in the 20 years before screening was introduced (1958 to 1977) with those from breast cancer diagnosed in the 20 years after the introduction of screening (1978 to 1997).[23] The study population consisted of 210,000 women between the ages of 20 and 69 years of age. The findings showed that among women aged 40 to 69 who were screened, there was significantly lower breast cancer mortality compared to those diagnosed in the earlier time period. Women in the same age range who were not exposed to screening had significantly higher breast cancer mortality. In the 20 to 39 age group, there was no significant difference in breast cancer mortality in 1978 to 1997 compared with 1958 to 1977. The researchers concluded that mammography screening contributed to the substantial reductions in breast cancer mortality among women over age 40.

Other studies also have shown benefits of mammography in younger as well as older women.[24] Gains in survival are perhaps a result of a high proportion of cancers being diagnosed and treated at more favorable stages as a result of early detection screening. Another benefit from screening is that it allows the individual a wider choice of treatment options.

An updated review of the Swedish trials extended the follow-up period and looked at the age-specific and trial-specific effects on breast cancer mortality.[25] The researchers concluded that there is a statistically significant reduction in breast cancer mortality, and the effect of breast screening on breast cancer mortality persists after long-term follow-up. In their opinion, the data affirm that screening mammography has a real but modest effect on mortality from breast cancer, although this effect varies by age. The reduction in breast cancer mortality is greatest among those 60 to 69 at entry to the study, and there were statistically significant effects in the age groups 50 to 59, 60 to 64, and 65 to 69. There was a small effect among those in the 50 to 54 age group. That is, the benefits of screening become statistically significant beginning at age 55. Among 55 to 64 year-old women, deaths among those who were screened were reduced by 27%. Deaths were reduced by 14% among those 45- to 54-year-olds who were screened. The conclusion that the advantageous effect of breast screening on breast cancer mortality persists after long-term follow-up directly challenges the Danish researchers' findings.

Concluding Thoughts

And the debate continues. The trials discussed here included approximately 500,000 women. Each study was designed to look at the potential benefits of mammography (e.g., survival) and potential drawbacks (e.g., no benefit in mortality reduction). For better or for worse, the findings from each of the trials have contributed to the ongoing debate about mammography's effectiveness among women of different ages. Many of the studies were criticized for their methodological flaws. Both proponents and opponents of mammography screening found evidence to support their viewpoint, both sides relying on the same data but drawing different conclusions. More studies are being conducted to assess the potential of the new breast cancer screening tools to reduce mortality. While the mammogram debate is far from settled, this leaves the individual woman in a position where she will have to make a decision to get screened or not based on her own perceived risks of breast cancer. The epidemiological studies and clinical trials are impersonal in that they rely on data from many individuals. An individual woman's decision is much more emotional and personal. Should I get screened? What are *my risks* of developing breast cancer over the next few years, and how will mammography help *me*?

CHAPTER EIGHT

Breast Cancer Treatment Options: Which Treatments Are the "Best"?

While the diagnosis of breast cancer can be devastating, this disease is not uniformly fatal, and there are some very effective treatment options widely available. Medical research has made, and continues to make, great strides in unlocking the secrets of breast cancer with new techniques for diagnosis, new treatment modalities, and advances in molecular genetics. There are many differences in its etiology and pathology, with some cases characterized by slow growth and other cases being highly aggressive. Breast tumors differ based on the expression of estrogen receptors (ERs), progesterone receptors (PRs), and human epidermal growth factor 2 (HER2) oncogene (i.e., a gene that has the potential to cause cancer). The type of treatment will be dictated by many factors, including patient characteristics, type of breast cancer, and hormone receptor status. The good news is there are so many options to consider. A "one-size-fits-all" approach is a thing of the past.

Cancer Staging

It is important to understand that breast cancer is not one entity. In order to determine the nature of the cancer, a staging system was developed to describe where a cancer is located, the size of the tumor, if or where it has spread, and whether it is affecting other parts of the body. Cancer is typically labeled in stages from I to IV, with IV being the most serious. Staging is an important indicator of the extent of cancer growth and is often crucial for identifying appropriate treatment options. It also helps physicians discern prognosis.

Most cancer staging systems include information about where the tumor is located in the body, the cell type (i.e., adenocarcinoma or squamous cell carcinoma), size of the tumor, whether the cancer has spread to nearby lymph nodes, and whether the cancer has spread to a different part of the body (i.e., metastasized). Although staging of a cancer is important, treatment options are often influenced by other factors such as age, ethnicity, and comorbid conditions. Not every woman with the same staging will receive the same treatment or will have the same prognosis.

Stage 0 indicates that abnormal cells are present, but the cancer is where it started (in situ) and hasn't spread. This is called carcinoma in situ (CIS). CIS is not cancer, but it could become cancer. Abnormal cells may be present, but they have not spread to nearby tissue. Ductal carcinoma in situ (DCIS) is an example of Stage 0 breast cancer. Overall, the relative five-year survival rate for Stage 0 cancer is 100%.

Stage I refers to a cancer that is small and has not spread. Stage 1 breast cancer is considered early breast cancer, with an overall five-year survival rate of 98%.

Stage II has two parts: Stage IIA refers to a cancerous tumor that has not spread to the lymph nodes. Stage IIB refers to a tumor that has spread to the axillary lymph nodes. Regarding breast cancer, the relative five-year survival rate for Stage IIA is 88% and 76% for Stage IIB.

Stage III also has two parts: Stage IIIA refers to a cancer that has spread to the lymph nodes. Stage IIIB refers to a cancer that has also spread to nearby tissues. Stage IIIA breast cancer has spread to the lymph nodes under the arm as well as to other lymph nodes. Stage IIIB breast cancer refers to a cancer that has spread to tissues near the breast (i.e., skin, chest wall), or the cancer has spread to lymph nodes inside the chest wall along the breast bone. Five-year survival for Stage IIIA breast cancer is 56% and 49% for Stage IIIB breast cancer.

Stage IV, the most serious staging, refers to a cancer that has spread to other parts of the body (i.e., bone, lung, liver, brain). Five-year survival is much lower than that for the other stages.

There also is a staging system that is used by cancer registries to describe a cancer. *In situ* refers to the presence of abnormal cells that have not spread to nearby tissue. *Localized* cancers refer to cancerous cells that are limited to the place where it started, with no sign that the cancer has spread. *Regional* refers to a cancer that has spread to nearby lymph nodes, tissues, or organs, and *distant* means that a cancer has spread to distant parts of the body. The last category, *unknown*, means that there is not enough information to determine the stage.

In addition to staging, the cancerous cells can be graded. Tumor grade provides a description based on how abnormal the tumor cells and the tumor tissue look under a microscope. Tumor grade is an indicator of how quickly a tumor is likely to grow and spread. A *well-differentiated* tumor is one in which the cells of the tumor and the organization of the tumor's tissue are close to those of normal cells and tissue. These tumors tend to grow and spread at a slower rate than tumors that are *undifferentiated* or *poorly differentiated*. Well-differentiated cancer cells look more like normal cells and tend to grow and spread more slowly than poorly differentiated or undifferentiated cancer cells. Undifferentiated cancer cells are very immature and "primitive" and do not look like cells in the tissue from which they arose. Poorly differentiated tumor cells also do not look like normal cells, as they tend to be disorganized under the microscope and grow and spread faster than Grade I tumors.

Tumors are graded as 1, 2, 3, or 4, depending on the amount of abnormality. In Grade 1 tumors, the tumor cells and the organization of the tumor tissue appear close to normal. These tumors tend to grow and spread slowly. In contrast, the cells and tissue of Grade 3 and Grade 4 tumors do not look like normal cells and tissue, and these tumors tend to grow rapidly and spread faster than tumors with a lower grade.[1]

Another cancer staging system used by most hospitals and medical centers as their main method for cancer reporting is the TNM system. In the TNM system, the "T" refers to the size and extent of the main tumor (i.e., the primary tumor); the "N" refers to the number of nearby lymph nodes that have cancerous cells; and the "M" refers to whether the cancer has metastasized.

Survival Issues

Breast cancer survival rates have increased substantially over the past decades, and much of the success in prolonging life after diagnosis can be attributed to advances in treatment. Survival is conventionally delineated by five-year survival rates, which refers to the average number of individuals who are still alive five years after diagnosis. It is important to stress, however, that survival rates are based on averages, and some women will live longer than others. In general, a lower stage rating and tumor grade implies a more favorable prognosis. A higher-grade cancer may grow and spread more quickly and may require immediate or more aggressive treatment. Survival depends on many factors, including the type of breast cancer, the size and location of the cancerous tumor, whether the cancer was diagnosed at an early or more advanced stage, and individual risk factors.

Since 1975, the breast cancer five-year relative survival rate in the United States has increased substantially for women in the major race/ethnic groups.

While there still remains a gap, especially for late-stage diagnoses, the racial/ethnic disparity seems to be narrowing. Based on the most recent data from the American Cancer Society, relative survival rates for women diagnosed with breast cancer are 91% after 5 years after diagnosis, 86% after 10 years, and 80% after 15 years.[2] The relative 5-year survival rate for women under age 50 years is 90.7%, and for women 50 years and older, the rate is 90.5%, essentially identical to that of younger women. Five-year survival rates are equally impressive when one looks at stage and tumor size; however, the five-year survival rate is only 27% among those with distant stage disease.

Among racial/ethnic groups, there are disparities in survival. As was discussed in chapter 6, the racial/ethnic disparity in survival reflects the later stage at diagnosis and poorer stage-specific survival in African American women, as well as higher rates of more aggressive, triple-negative breast cancer among women in this racial/ethnic group.

It is important to explain that long-term survival rates are based on the experience of women diagnosed and treated many years ago and may not reflect the most recent advances in early detection and treatment. We now know so much more about breast cancer pathogenesis, which has led to very impressive advances in breast cancer treatment and survival. Depending on the stage and type of breast cancer, a treatment plan can be designed to yield the most positive outcome for the individual.

Breast Cancer Treatment Options: One Size Does Not Fit All

Given that there are different stages of breast cancer and different types of breast cancer, there is not one specific treatment that is "best" for all breast cancer patients. Each option has its own specific advantages and disadvantages, and each has side effects, ranging from mild to more serious. Often, different types of treatment will be used in combination simultaneously or sequentially. Which treatment or treatments are deemed the most appropriate will often depend on a number of factors, including the tumor size, histologic type, lymph node status, biomarkers (i.e., measurable parameters in tissues, cells, or fluids), stage of the disease, hormone receptor status, and personal characteristics of the individual. For example, most women with early-stage breast cancer will have some type of surgery, often combined with other treatments to reduce the risk of recurrence. Those who have metastatic breast cancer are primarily treated with systemic therapies such as chemotherapy, targeted therapy, or hormonal therapy.

While the clinical parameters of the disease usually dictate the type of treatment, an individual's input is very important. Individual patients differ in the importance they place on the risks and benefits of treatment. Self-image, lifestyle, and quality of life needs are important considerations that must be taken into account in the decision-making. Whatever the treatment, be it surgery, radiation, chemotherapy, and/or hormonal treatment, the goal is the same: to kill the cancer cells. Surgery and radiation are local treatments in that they are directed at one area of the breast, whereas chemotherapy and hormonal therapy are systemic treatments that target the entire body. These treatments may be given individually or in some combination, either simultaneously or sequentially, depending on a host of factors.

Advances in Surgical Treatment of Breast Cancer

Surgery is often the first line of treatment for many of the solid tumors, which include cancers of the brain, ovary, and breast. The primary goals of breast cancer surgery are to remove the tumor and determine its stage. In some cases, surgical excision may be sufficient without other forms of treatment. In other instances, surgical resection is followed by a course of radiation and/or chemotherapy.

Over the decades, changes in breast cancer treatment protocol have made treating breast cancer with surgery much less invasive without jeopardizing survival. In the 19th century and well into the 20th century, a radical mastectomy was essentially the only surgical option for breast cancer regardless of type or size of the tumor. In 1804, Japanese surgeon Seishu Hanaoka performed the world's first mastectomy under general anesthesia, but it was Dr. William Halsted who is credited with scientifically describing this type of breast surgery.[3] In 1894, Dr. Halsted published his work on radical mastectomy that was based on the 50 cases he operated on at the Johns Hopkins Hospital between 1889 and 1894. He touted a local recurrence rate of just 7%, a rate that was unmatched by his peers. Halsted's technique prevailed for 70 years, and, based on his work, the surgical standard of care for breast cancer was to perform a radical mastectomy. In this procedure, the entire breast as well as the underlying chest muscle (including pectoralis major and pectoralis minor) and lymph nodes of the axilla were removed. Halsted and others believed that the most important pathway for breast cancer dissemination was through the lymphatic ducts; therefore, chances of cure would be increased if the lymph nodes of the axilla were removed along with breast tissue. At that time, it was also considered anatomically impossible to do a complete axillary dissection without removing the pectoralis muscles.[4] While survival after radical mastectomy was much higher than that for untreated patients, subsequent side effects were not insignificant, including restriction of arm movement and chronic pain.

In 1948, the modified radical mastectomy, which spared the pectoralis muscles, was introduced by Drs. Patey and Dyson from Middlesex Hospital in London.[5] They developed a procedure that preserved the pectoralis major muscle (a large muscle in the upper chest, fanning across the chest from the shoulder to the breastbone) and compared their operation with the standard radical mastectomy. They found no difference in survival or local recurrence rates between the two groups.[6] The modified radical mastectomy was somewhat less disfiguring than the more aggressive radical mastectomy.

In 1972, Dr John Madden and colleagues devised a technique to preserve both pectoral major muscles (today commonly referred to as the "pecs").[7] In their procedure, the entire breast, including the breast tissue, skin, areola and nipple and most of the underarm (axillary) lymph nodes, is removed, but both the pectoralis major and the pectoralis minor muscles are preserved. Since the chest muscles are left intact, there is no hollow in the chest, which is the case when a radical mastectomy is performed. The Madden-modified radical mastectomy was shown to be equally effective and less disfiguring than a radical mastectomy.

In the 1960s, the simple mastectomy was developed by Kennedy and Miller, based on indications that radical mastectomy was not always necessary in women with breast cancer.[8] This procedure involved removal of the breast, but neither the pectoralis muscles nor the axillary lymph nodes are removed. Findings from research studies helped convince oncologists and surgeons that the simple mastectomy is equally effective to the more radical surgical procedures. In particular, Drs. Kaae and Johansen[9] compared simple mastectomy plus postoperative radiotherapy with extended radical mastectomy plus radiotherapy and found that overall survival rates were similar in both. With new evidence that breast-conserving surgery was equally effective clinically, and certainly less disfiguring and mutilating, performing radical and modified radical mastectomies fell out of favor.

Toward the end of the 20th century, less aggressive surgical approaches were introduced. In 1991, Drs. Toth and Lappert devised a skin-sparing mastectomy for breast cancer treatment in order to facilitate breast reconstruction. In a skin-sparing mastectomy, the surgeon removes only the skin of the nipple, areola, and the original biopsy scar and removes the breast tissue through the small opening that is created. Many women choose this type of mastectomy so as to have breast reconstruction at the time of the mastectomy. Importantly, the risk of local cancer recurrence with this type of mastectomy is the same as with other types of mastectomies. However, this procedure might not be suitable for those who have large tumors or tumors that are close to the surface of the skin.

The removal of the nipples was often cosmetically upsetting to many women, which led to the nipple-sparing mastectomy, a variation of the skin-sparing mastectomy in which the breast tissue is removed, but the breast skin and nipple are left in place. The nipple-sparing mastectomy did much to alleviate concerns about not having the breast look "normal." While the technique of nipple-sparing mastectomy was originally described in the 1960s, it was not widely performed. In 1999, an article published in the *New England Journal of Medicine* was one of the first to document the benefits of this procedure, which included the potential to reduce postmastectomy deformity, better breast shape after reconstruction, less residual scarring, and greater patient satisfaction.[10] This and other studies provided empirical evidence of and support to the nipple-sparing mastectomy's acceptance by patients and surgeons. A meta-analysis published in 2015 compared overall survival, disease-free survival, and local recurrence in breast cancer patients who had nipple-sparing mastectomy and found no significant differences in these outcomes compared to women undergoing modified radical mastectomy or skin-sparing mastectomy.[11]

Some women who have a mastectomy also elect to have breast reconstruction using autologous tissue (a person's own skin and tissues), implants, or both either at the time of the mastectomy or thereafter. Breast reconstruction also can be done many months or even years after breast surgery. The objective is to provide symmetry of the breasts and to have the individual feel more comfortable about her appearance. Reconstruction will depend on the type of mastectomy performed, skin and muscle condition, breast size, and postoperative treatment. For example, women who will have postmastectomy radiation would not be candidates for reconstruction at the time of mastectomy.

Surgeons as well as women with breast cancer have rightfully questioned whether it is "better" to have a mastectomy or opt for breast-conserving surgery. Both have been shown to be effective therapies for invasive breast cancer; however, type of tumor, size, age, and other factors will have to be taken into account when making a decision about which course of surgical treatment would be best for the specific patient. The definitive answer to this question was based on the work of Dr. Bernard Fisher, who conducted pioneering research that showed that early-stage breast cancers could be treated with more simple surgical procedures and that subsequent treatment with chemotherapy or hormonal drugs could increase survival time.

Fighting fierce resistance from his colleagues, Dr. Fisher was steadfast in his belief that less invasive procedures could be as good as the more radical ones. In his opinion, the radical surgeries made no biological sense. In order to obtain the data he needed to prove his point, he conducted a clinical trial to test his hypothesis. A total of 1,765 patients were divided into three groups: radical mastectomy, simple mastectomy, and lumpectomy followed by radiation. Lumpectomy is the surgical removal of the tumor and some of the normal tissue surrounding it (not the entire breast), whereas partial mastectomy is the removal of the cancerous part of the breast tissue and some normal tissue around it. While lumpectomy is technically a form of partial mastectomy, more tissue is removed in partial mastectomy than in lumpectomy.

The findings from Fisher's studies showed empirically that those who received the radical mastectomy had more disability and disfigurement, but did not have longer survival than those who received a lumpectomy. To the surprise of many physicians and surgeons, there was no difference in cancer recurrence, metastasis, or death rates among the different types of procedures.[12] This study and others like it helped shift the paradigm away from the radical mastectomy to much less invasive surgical procedures. Dr Fisher and his group also convincingly showed that hormone drug therapy with Tamoxifen could reduce cancer recurrence when administered after surgery. This "game-changing" drug will be discussed in a later section.

Since Dr. Fisher's pioneering work, many more studies have been conducted to assess the benefits and limitations of mastectomy and breast-conserving surgery (i.e., lumpectomy or partial mastectomy).[13,14] A 2010 meta-analysis that compared skin-sparing mastectomy to conventional mastectomy showed no difference in local recurrence between the two procedures,[15] and a successive large retrospective review of 1,810 patients also demonstrated no significant difference in local, regional, or systemic recurrence rates between the two procedures at a median follow-up of 53 months.[16]

Based on the evidence, breast-conserving surgery followed by a course of radiation became the norm for those who did not have advanced cancer. Clinical trials and observational studies found that survival among women with Stage I or II breast cancer who had breast-conserving surgery followed by radiation or mastectomy was the same as for those who had other types of mastectomies performed. And some studies suggested that breast-conserving surgery conferred improved survival and reduced recurrence rates with breast-conserving surgery.[17,18] Further, the risk of complications was much lower among those who had breast-conserving surgery.[19]

For some women, however, breast-conserving surgery is not an option. Women who have had prior radiation therapy to the breast or chest wall, who are diagnosed with inflammatory breast cancer, who have diffuse suspicious or malignant-appearing microcalcifications, or have tumors larger than 5 cm should have a mastectomy. Those who are younger than age 35 or who are premenopausal with known *BRCA1/2* mutations should have a mastectomy.

For those for whom breast-conserving surgery is an option, research findings are reassuring. A large trial conducted in Europe, The European Organization for Research and Treatment of Cancer 10801 trial, found no significant difference in the 20-year survival rate among women with Stage 1 or Stage 2 breast cancer between those who had breast-conserving surgery and radiation and those who had a modified radical mastectomy.[20]

There are women at high risk of developing breast cancer who make a proactive decision to have a prophylactic mastectomy in which one or both breasts are removed in hopes of preventing or reducing the risk of breast cancer. For example, if a woman has had one breast removed because of a cancer diagnosis, and has the *BRCA1* or *BRCA2* mutation, she may decide to have the other unaffected breast removed. Women with a strong family history of breast cancer may elect to have a prophylactic mastectomy in hopes of reducing the risk of breast cancer. In 2013, the actress Angelina Jolie, who has a family history of breast cancer, famously went public with her very private decision to have a preemptive double mastectomy to reduce her risk of developing breast cancer. She said she did this because she had the *BRCA1* mutation, which increased the odds of her developing breast or ovarian cancer. Her decision, and more importantly her desire to go public with it, did much to make women aware of what the *BRCA1* and *BRCA2* mutations are and what options are available even in the absence of the diagnosis of breast cancer. The number of women opting for a double prophylactic mastectomy increased during the 2000s.[21] Yet, there are pros and cons of elective a prophylactic mastectomy,[22] and the decision should be made in consultation with one's doctor.

Over the past decades, the empirical evidence from studies of various surgical options for treating breast cancer led to many viable options that the surgeon and patient can consider. Findings show conclusively that partial mastectomy is not necessarily superior to breast-conserving surgery and that uniformly performing a mastectomy may not necessarily be the most appropriate surgical treatment of choice. Today, surgical options range from simple or total mastectomy to partial mastectomy, lumpectomy (also known as breast-conservation surgery), nipple-sparing subcutaneous mastectomy, and skin-sparing mastectomy. Another procedure similar to lumpectomy is the quadrantectomy, which essentially is a partial mastectomy that involves removing more breast tissue than in a lumpectomy, but the surgeon still leaves most of the breast tissue intact. Given the various surgical options available, having a frank discussion with one's surgeon is so important before making any surgical decision.

Advances in Radiation Treatment for Breast Cancer

Radiotherapy (RT), used alone or in association with different treatments, has been used for treating a wide range of malignancies for more than 100 years. Thanks to the experiment conducted by Wilhelm Conrad Roentgen in 1895 in which he recorded the shadow of his wife's hand and rings on a photographic plate (see the following image), the use of x-ray treatment was ushered in. Therapeutic uses of x-rays in cancer rapidly followed when it became apparent that rapidly growing cells, such as cancer cells, are more susceptible to the effects of RT than normal cells.

In the early 20th century, the idea of using radioactive elements to treat cancer was spurred by the discoveries of radium and polonium by Marie and Pierre Curie; however, a lack of knowledge on the properties and mechanism of actions of RT were not well understood, including unintended side effects (some quite serious) from the radiation. Early use of

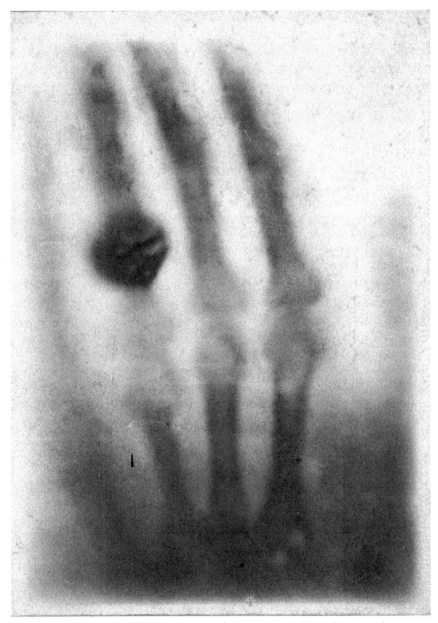

The bones of a hand with a ring on one finger, viewed through x-ray. Photoprint from radiograph by W. K. Röntgen, 1895. (Wellcome Library no. 32971i)

RT as a treatment for breast cancer included placing low-energy cathode ray tubes or radium-filled glass tubes in close proximity to the breast tumor. More often than not, this method caused extensive damage to normal tissue (i.e., skin burns). Also, early RT was limited in that devices could only produce low x-ray energies, which could not penetrate deep into tissues.

Over the course of time, knowledge about cancer biology and how radiation affects human tissues on the cellular level led to the development of more powerful RT techniques and helped clarify the benefits and harms of RT.[23] Experimentation with low-dose rate radium treatments conducted over the course of several weeks was the foundation for fractionation for external beam radiotherapy (XRT). A shift to XRT, in which fractions are delivered over weeks or months using relatively small doses of radiation, helped preserve normal tissues while killing malignant tissues. As new radioactive isotopes and radiation techniques were discovered, the use, safety, and value of RT became clearer. New techniques enabled the delivery of a higher, targeted dose of RT to tumors, making possible the treatment of deep tumors while limiting side effects, such as excessive radiation to normal tissues surrounding the malignant tumor.

In the 1970s and 1980s, computer-assisted accelerator for protons was successfully applied to treat a different kind of tumors, and by the end of the 1990s, even more sophisticated modalities were introduced, including intensity-modulated radiation therapy (IMRT), brachytherapy (use of radioactive material in the form of a seed, pellet, wire, or capsule that is implanted in the body using a needle or catheter—this treatment is most commonly used to treat prostate cancer), stereotactic radiation therapy (a nonsurgical radiation therapy that can deliver precisely targeted radiation in fewer high-dose treatments than traditional therapy), cyber-knife therapy (a procedure that delivers high doses of precisely targeted radiation beams), gamma knife therapy (a form of stereotactic radiosurgery used to treat abnormalities in the brain), proton beam therapy (a type of radiation therapy that uses protons rather than x-rays to treat cancer), the introduction of the adaptive RT (ART) (a type of radiation therapy process where treatment is adapted to account for changes in a patient's internal anatomy), image-guided radiotherapy (IGRT) (a type of radiation therapy that uses high-quality images taken before each radiation therapy treatment session so as to improve definition, localization, and monitoring of tumor position, size, and shape before and during treatment), and accelerated partial breast irradiation (APBI) for low-risk patients (a type of radiation therapy that treats only the lumpectomy bed plus a 1 to 2 cm margin, rather than the whole breast). The use of APBI is an example of delivering internal radiation therapy to target the tumor while limiting radiation exposure to normal tissue and organs surrounding the tumor.

The MammoSite Radiation Therapy System™ (RTS) is another type of accelerated breast radiation treatment that was approved by the FDA in 2002. The procedure can be used after lumpectomy and relies on a balloon brachytherapy method that directly targets the lumpectomy cavity where the cancer is most likely to recur, sparing healthy tissues and organs from the damaging effects of radiation.[24] RST treatments are done twice a day for five consecutive days as compared with a course of six or seven weeks for external beam radiation. Women who have highly confined lesions and who have involvement of only three or fewer lymph nodes would be the "best" candidates for this type of RT. A 2014 study of over 100 women who underwent MammoSite balloon brachytherapy showed excellent tumor control over a median follow-up of 5.5 years.[25] However, complications after MammoSite brachytherapy have been reported to occur at significantly higher rates when compared to whole breast RT.[26] Thus, a discussion with one's physician is necessary before decisions about using this type of APBI.

Over the years, numerous studies have been conducted to document the potential benefits and harms of RT for breast cancer treatment. For some types of breast cancer, RT only is sufficient. For other types, RT is used in conjunction with chemotherapy or hormone therapy. Numerous studies and trials conducted around the world have shown long-term benefits of RT, including reducing the risk of cancer recurrence and overall survival. For example, whole-breast irradiation and accelerated partial breast irradiation are associated with low rates of cancer recurrence in women with early-stage breast cancer for more than 5 years to more than 10 years.[27] Other studies show that use of RT after either breast-conserving surgery or mastectomy in node-positive patients not only reduces local recurrence but also improves long-term survival.[28] RT is also used to treat the symptoms of advanced breast cancer, especially when the cancer has spread to the central nervous system or bones.

While major advances have been made in RT, emphasis now is on refining treatments to provide more options for patients, such as shorter courses of individualized, targeted radiation therapy. As the above discussion illustrates, many RT options are now available. RT may be administered as external beam radiation (the beam is highly focused and targets the cancerous area for two to three minutes) or internal beam radiation such as brachytherapy (radioactive materials are placed in the body), or a combination of both. Choice of therapy will depend on the type, stage, and location of the tumor as well as patient characteristics. For individuals with advanced breast disease, for example, postmastectomy radiation is a well-established course of treatment. For those with early breast cancer, however, the consensus is not as clear. The most important predictor of use of RT after surgery is the extent of axillary nodal disease, especially since axillary nodes are usually the initial site of metastases in the majority of breast cancer patients. Overall, it is estimated that about two-thirds of all cancer patients receive some type of RT as part of their treatment for cancer.[29] RT is referred to as an adjuvant therapy, which means a treatment that is given in addition to the primary (initial) treatment (i.e., surgery). The selection of the type of adjuvant therapy is based on patient characteristics such as age, ethnicity, tumor size, histologic type, hormone receptor status, and other biomarkers (i.e., measurable parameters in tissues, cells, or fluids). Whereas localized adjuvant treatment (i.e., RT) focuses on a specific part of the body, systemic adjuvant therapy acts on the whole body. Systemic treatments include chemotherapy and hormonal therapy.

Chemotherapy (Adjuvant Systemic Therapy)

Chemotherapy, the treatment of cancer with drugs, is used in addition to surgery and/or RT in an effort to kill dividing cancer cells and prevent them from multiplying. These agents are given intravenously or orally, and usually multiple combinations of drugs can be used. Chemotherapy drugs are divided into several categories based on how they affect specific chemical substances within cancer cells, which cellular activities or processes the drug interferes with, and which specific phases of the cell cycle the drug affects. Some work directly on DNA to prevent cancer cells from reproducing. Some interfere with DNA growth. Sometimes chemotherapy is given before surgery to help shrink the tumor (neoadjuvant chemotherapy). Whereas neoadjuvant therapies are delivered before the main treatment to help reduce the size of a tumor or kill cancer cells that have spread, adjuvant therapies are delivered after the primary treatment to destroy remaining cancer cells.

Many factors have to be taken into account before chemotherapy is prescribed. The choice of chemotherapy is dependent on many factors, including size of tumor and grade, number of lymph nodes involved, presence of estrogen or progesterone receptors, presence of HER2 overexpression, and age of the individual. HER2-directed therapy is a critical component of the adjuvant treatment of HER2-positive breast cancer. The availability of HER2 targeted agents (i.e., paclitaxel, trastuzumab, pertuzumab, docetaxel, carboplatin) has dramatically changed for the better the prognosis of patients with HER2-positive breast cancer. The choice will be dependent on the biology of the disease as determined by hormone receptor status.

Adjuvant chemotherapy is standard for patients with triple-negative breast cancer and either a tumor size >0.5 cm or lymph node involvement (regardless of tumor size).[30] Women with very small (1 to 3 mm) node-negative tumors generally do not need chemotherapy. In an effort to help oncologists decide on the most appropriate adjuvant chemotherapy regimen, the Oncotype Dx21-Gene Recurrence Score is widely used in decision-making. A high score indicates that the woman would more likely benefit from adjuvant chemotherapy, and a low score indicates that chemotherapy is probably not necessary.[31] The score is independent of an individual's age and tumor size.

The benefits of adjuvant chemotherapy in early breast cancer have been demonstrated in a large meta-analysis.[32] There are many excellent chemotherapy regimens available, the choice of which will depend on the clinical and pathological manifestation of the type of breast cancer a woman has. One or more drugs may be prescribed in combination, depending on the specifics of the individual's breast cancer.

Endocrine (Hormonal) Therapy

The growth of some breast cancers is sensitive or dependent on certain female hormones, estrogen in particular. Overall, ER-positive breast cancer is the most common type of breast cancer diagnosed. Breast tissue is analyzed to determine if the cancer cells have estrogen or progesterone receptors. ERs and PRs (also called PgRs) may be found in breast cancer cells. Breast cancer cells that have ERs are called ER-positive breast cancer, and breast cancer cells that have progesterone receptors are called PR-positive breast cancer. If the cells do not have either of these two receptors, the cancer is called ER/PR-negative. Breast tumors that lack both estrogen and progesterone receptors are called hormone receptor negative (HR-negative). Endocrine therapy is recommended for most patients with HR-positive disease.

The more ERs that are present, the more likely it is that antiestrogen therapy would be prescribed. The theory is that if there were less estrogen in the body, the hormone receptors would receive fewer growth signals so that cancer overgrowth can be controlled or stopped. Estrogen promotes the growth of breast cancer cells, but there are ways of medically blocking the effects of estrogen on these cells. Hormonal therapy, also called endocrine therapy, is designed to control the growth of hormone receptor positive breast cancer cells by blocking the receptors, lowering the hormone levels, or eliminating receptors. However, tumors that do not have hormone receptors do not respond to hormone therapy. Antiestrogen therapy is not as effective in cancers that have few if any ERs.

Individuals whose cancers are progesterone-receptor positive may also respond to antiestrogen therapy. If both estrogen and progesterone receptors are present, the chance of responding to antiestrogen therapy is high (~70%). For those who are estrogen-receptor positive only or progesterone-receptor positive only, the likelihood of responding to antiestrogen therapy is much less (~33%). And if neither receptor is positive, the odds of responding to this type of therapy are quite low (~10%).

Over the past decades, there have been remarkable advances in hormonal therapies for breast cancer. Drugs designed to block the effects of hormones or lower the hormonal levels in the blood have increased the survival of women whose breast cancer is hormone dependent. For example, selective estrogen receptor modulators (SERMs) are powerful agents that not only act against the effects of estrogen in breast tissue but also act like estrogen in other tissues. Probably the best known SERM is tamoxifen (brand name Nolvadex), an antiestrogen that has become one of the world's best-selling hormonal breast cancer drugs.

First synthesized in 1962 within a project to develop a contraceptive pill in the pharmaceutical laboratories of ICI (now part of AstraZeneca), it was designed to act as an antiestrogen, but the compound stimulated, rather than suppressed, ovulation in women.[33] Those working on the drug then switched to investigate its potential for use in breast cancer cases. In the 1980s, small clinical trials showed that tamoxifen was useful as an adjuvant to surgery and chemotherapy in the early stages of breast cancer. Subsequent trials demonstrated that it could prevent breast cancer occurrence or re-occurrence in women at high risk of breast cancer.

Tamoxifen, hailed as a pioneering drug, is now widely prescribed for the treatment of early and advanced HR-positive breast cancer in both pre- and postmenopausal women. Studies show convincingly that taking tamoxifen for at least 5 years reduces the rate of breast cancer recurrence by 40 to 50% and reduces breast cancer mortality by one-third over the course of 15 years.[34] Further research has shown that taking tamoxifen for 10 years is beneficial, so clinical practice guidelines now recommend consideration of a course of tamoxifen for 10 years.[35] A note of caution: there are some women, particularly those with early-stage breast cancer, who receive tamoxifen and develop a resistance within 2 to 5 years.

Raloxifene (brand name Evista) is another SERM that has been shown to be effective in women with ER-positive breast cancer. Marketed as a medication used to prevent and treat osteoporosis in postmenopausal women and those on glucocorticoids, it is also used to reduce the risk of breast cancer in postmenopausal women. In the Multiple Outcomes of Raloxifene (MORE) clinical trial, raloxifene decreased the risk of all types of breast cancer by 62%, invasive breast cancer by 72%, and invasive ER-positive breast cancer by 84%.[36] Conversely, it does not reduce the risk of ER-negative breast cancer.

There are differences between tamoxifen and raloxifene in terms of the effect on the uterus. Tamoxifen has an estrogen-like effect, while raloxifene acts as an estrogen antagonist. Unlike tamoxifen, raloxifene has no risk of uterine hyperplasia or endometrial cancer. Tamoxifen has been associated with endometrial hyperplasia, fibroids, polyps, thrombosis, and endometrial tumors, as well as other side effects, including hot flashes, vaginal discharge, menstrual irregularities, sexual dysfunction, and blood clots.[37] Use of tamoxifen has been associated with a slightly increased risk of cataracts, although this appears to be a rare problem. There was some concern that tamoxifen may cause or worsen depression; however, a large five-year study that included over 11,000 women found no increased rates of depression among those taking tamoxifen.[38] Although longer treatment with tamoxifen has the potential to increase the risk of adverse effects, the thinking is that reduction in breast cancer mortality associated with longer treatment outweighs those risks. Common side effects of raloxifene include hot flashes, vaginal dryness, and mild leg cramps.

It is important to understand that hormone therapy for breast cancer probably will be different in premenopausal and postmenopausal women. For example, among postmenopausal women, long-term use of tamoxifen may double the risk of endometrial cancer. For these women, it might be useful to consider treatment with an aromatase inhibitor.

Aromatase Inhibitors

Aromatase inhibitors (AIs) are a class of medicines that work by interfering with the body's ability to produce estrogen from androgens by suppressing aromatase enzyme activity, thus limiting the supply of estrogen that helps promote the growth of some breast cancers. AIs are only prescribed for postmenopausal women. AIs have a limited ability to reduce circulating estrogen in premenopausal women. Unlike postmenopausal women, premenopausal women have a large amount of aromatase substrate present in the ovary.

There are three main AIs: Letrozole (brand name Femara), Anastrazole (brand name Arimidex), and Exemestane (brand name Aromasin). These are third-generation AIs that have largely replaced tamoxifen as the preferred treatment for HR-positive breast cancer in postmenopausal women. Letrozole was approved by the FDA in 2005 for postmenopausal women in early-stage or late-stage hormone-sensitive breast cancer who had completed 5 years of tamoxifen treatment. A large clinical trial showed that this AI reduced the risk of breast cancer recurrence and spread more than tamoxifen alone.[39] The trial was actually stopped 2.5 years before the planned 5 years of study because the findings were so compelling. By stopping the study, however, some important questions would not be answered, such as the following: To what extent does Letrozole promote actual survival? How long should women take the drug? What are the consequences of long-term use? The most common treatment-related adverse events reported are hot flushes, nausea, and hair thinning.

Anastrazole has been shown to improve survival for postmenopausal women with advanced breast cancer. A large-scale clinical trial found that Anastrazole was better than tamoxifen in postmenopausal women diagnosed with early-stage ER-positive breast cancer and/or progesterone-receptor positive breast cancer. Anastrazole reduced the risk of breast cancer recurrence by

17% more than tamoxifen alone and decreased the chances of breast cancer developing in the other breast by almost 80%.[40] Exemestane is indicated for the treatment of advanced breast cancer in postmenopausal women who have received tamoxifen previously and whose disease has progressed following this therapy. Anastrozole, exemestane, and letrozole have largely replaced tamoxifen as the preferred treatment for HR-positive breast cancer in postmenopausal women, by far the most prevalent among breast cancer patients.

A logical question one might ask is, Which AI is "better" or "best"? Studies have shown that there is no clear advantage to one AI versus another at the present time, and oncologists often select an AI depending on the type of adjuvant strategy they wish to use based on the characteristics of the patient and tumor.

The benefits of AIs include no increase in uterine cancers or thromboembolic events, as is observed with tamoxifen, with the exception of hot flushes. However, women taking AIs are more likely to complain of symptoms related to estrogen deprivation, and they must be monitored for osteoporosis, as AIs can decrease bone density. Clinical trials are ongoing to assess the optimal timing and duration of AIs.

Today, there are so many options for treating breast cancer, and no one treatment should be considered the "best." So much depends on the type of breast cancer, hormone receptor status, pre- or postmenopausal status, and other factors. It is not unusual to change treatments or combine treatments. For example, an individual could take tamoxifen for two or three years followed by treatment with an aromatase inhibitor for two or three years. Some women may take an aromatase inhibitor every day for five years, instead of tamoxifen. Other women may receive additional treatment with an aromatase inhibitor after five years of tamoxifen. The objective is to find the most appropriate treatment for the individual at a specific point in time.

Biological Therapy (Immunotherapy)/Targeted Therapy

Just as one's immune system defends the body against infections, it can also be the body's natural defense against cancer. New biological therapies use naturally occurring, normal proteins to repair, stimulate, and increase the body's ability to fight infections and cancer. Whereas chemotherapy uses chemical substances to treat cancer, biological therapy uses living organisms, substances derived from organisms, or laboratory-made versions of those substances to stimulate the body's immune system to act against cancer cells. Tailored or targeted therapy based on the presence or absence of receptors for estrogen, progesterone, and HER2 is the basis for biological targeted therapy.

The main targeted therapy used in breast cancer treatment is trastuzumab (brand name Herceptin), a monoclonal antibody that reduces the risk of breast cancer recurrence in women with HER2-positive breast cancer. HER2 is a key protein in regulating cell growth. An overexpression of HER2 causes an increased growth and reproduction, often resulting in more aggressive breast cancer with significantly shortened disease-free episodes and survival rates. In 2006, trastuzumab was approved as part of the adjuvant therapy for women with early-stage HER2-positive breast cancer. This drug works only against breast cancers that make too much of the HER2 protein. Simplistically put, trastuzumab attaches to the HER2 receptors on the surface of breast cancer cells and stops them from dividing and growing. Approximately 15 to 20% of breast cancer patients are affected by HER2 protein overexpression.[41]

Clinical trials have shown that trastuzumab significantly improves overall survival and disease-free survival in women with HER2-positive early breast cancer, but long-term follow-up data are needed.[42] In some cases, women develop resistance to trastuzumab, which leads to a recurrence or progression of the cancer. Also, a potentially serious side effect of taking trastuzumab is cardiotoxicity, which means that those taking the drug should have their heart monitored before and during treatment. Other less serious side effects include fever, chills, weakness, diarrhea, and nausea.

Several new drugs, pertuzumab (brand name Perjeta), docetaxel (brand name Taxotere), and capecitabine (brand name Xeloda), as well as new experimental compounds (i.e., tucatinib—development codes ARRY-380 and ONT-380) are being studied to be used in patients with HER2-positive metastatic breast cancer. Some would work in combination with trastuzumab or if trastuzumab is no longer working to achieve progression-free survival and overall survival. Tucatinib, in particular, is one of the most promising new drugs for women with Stage IV HER2-positive breast cancer. In trials, this drug nearly tripled one-year progression-free survival (33% vs 12%) and nearly doubled the two-year overall survival (45% vs 27%) in women with HER2-positive metastatic breast cancer.[43] However, at this time, no single regimen is considered the standard of care. That being said, these developments represent substantial progress in the treatment options for HER2-positive patients.

Women with HER2-negative advanced breast cancer will require different treatment modalities. Several international trials have tested the effectiveness of several drugs to increase progression-free survival and overall survival. For example, Ribociclib (brand name Kisqali), an antineoplastics that acts to prevent, inhibit, or halt the development of a tumor, is used in combination with letrozole in patients before or after menopause with hormone receptor positive, HER2-negative advanced or metastatic breast cancer. Fulvestrant (brand name Faslodex) also is being used to treat HR-positive metastatic breast cancer in postmenopausal women with disease progression as well as HR-positive, HER2-negative advanced breast cancer.

Research continues to provide information about the best combination of adjuvant therapy strategies. Ongoing studies are focusing on the identification of molecular markers that could be used to predict which patients would benefit the most from specific treatment regimens. Some women are at higher risk for the return or spread of cancer, although the reasons for this are not clear. It is difficult to explain why one patient stays cancer-free after treatment while another does not. There are several factors that probably contribute to recurrence and/or poor survival, including tumor size, involvement of lymph nodes, histological type of the cancer, and a woman's personal risk factors, which will dictate not only the type of treatment but also the likelihood of cancer recurrence.

Cryoablation/Cryotherapy

In addition to the pharmacological options, new techniques and approaches to treating breast cancer are available. Ablation of small tumors by cryoablation (the destruction of cancer cells through freezing) shows promise in treating women with low-risk breast cancers: The tumor is probed using an ultrasound-guided electric probe. The tip of the probe is chilled with argon gas to form an ice ball around the tumor, and cycles of freezing and thawing are performed to cause tumor cell death. Cryoablation therapy is performed without general anesthesia and in some cases can even be done in the physician's office. While it has yet to become an established treatment for breast cancer, studies are underway to assess the effectiveness of cryoablation as a primary treatment for breast cancer without surgical lumpectomy.

Great Reasons for Hope

With the advances in early cancer detection and treatment, the prognosis for most women diagnosed with breast cancer is excellent. The earlier the cancer is detected, the better the chances of recovery and survival. Treatment options are proliferating not just for early-stage breast cancer, but for advanced metastatic cancer as well. What should have been made clear in this chapter is that there is no treatment option that is the "right" or "only" one. Treatment will vary depending on a number of factors, including the histological type of the cancer, the stage, tumor size and location, how fast the cancer cells are growing (tests can measure how fast the cancer cells are dividing and how different they are compared to normal breast cells), lymph node involvement, whether the tumor is dependent on hormones and if so which ones, the individual's age and menopausal status, and her overall health status. Neoadjuvant and adjuvant therapies are tailored to the individual's situation and could include chemotherapy, biological therapy, and/or endocrine therapy. Almost all of the adjuvant therapies have short-and long-term side effects, some of which can be serious. Therefore, each individual must weigh the risks and benefits of the treatment options before deciding on the type or types of treatment modalities.

Most women diagnosed with breast cancer go on to live healthy and active lives. My mother lived over 15 active years after her diagnosis. In fact, after mastectomy and in her early 60s, she climbed not only the Himalayas but also the Peruvian Andes. When her cancer recurred in her late 60s, refusing to let her disease get the best of her, she managed to hike in the ruins of Petra (Jordan) with her daughter and granddaughter in between chemotherapy treatments!

Key Events in Breast Cancer Detection and Treatment

A Timeline through the Ages

Before Common Era (BCE)

- Egyptian papyri dating from 3500 BCE describe conditions of the breast consistent with what probably was breast disease, including cancer.

- Hippocrates (460 to 370 BCE) described breast cancer as a humoral disease characterized by an excess of black bile from breast tumors. If not treated, Hippocrates wrote that the tumor would harden and eventually rupture, releasing the black fluid into the rest of the body.

- Fourth-century BCE physicians described carcinoma, which referred to swellings that appear to be malignant or nonhealing swellings, or ulcerous formation.

Pre–Middle Age/Dark Age (Pre–15th Century)

- Galen (131 to 203 CE) provided a detailed description of abnormal growth in the breast. He believed that breast cancer was caused by accumulation of black bile formed in the liver (i.e., humoral theory). He suggested several treatment options, including a form of lumpectomy to remove the breast mass. (NOTE: There was no anesthesia at the time.)

- In the 1st century, Roman physicians routinely and crudely excised affected breasts with a hot cautery. In some cases, the pectoralia muscles were removed.

Age of Enlightenment (1715 to 1789)

- René Descartes (1596 to 1650) proposed the lymphatic theory for the origin of breast cancer, contradicting the prevailing humoral theory.
- Seventeenth-century physicians proposed absurd (in hindsight) theories for the cause of breast cancer (i.e., pus-filled inflammations, "vigorous" sex, depressive mental disorders).
- Henri Le Dran (1685 to 1770) and Claude-Nicolas Le Cat (1700 to 1768) advocated that surgery was the only way to treat breast cancer to prevent metastasis (metastasis theory).

Victorian Age (19th Century) into the 20th Century

- Rudolph Virchow (1821 to 1902) demonstrated that tumors were composed of cells.
- William Halsted (1852 to 1922) performed the first radical mastectomy, which remained the standard surgical operation to treat breast cancer well into the 20th century.
- Thomas Beatson (1848 to 1933) postulated that breast cancer is hormonal-dependent. He is considered to be the father of antihormonal treatment of breast cancer.
- Wilhelm Conrad Röentgen (1845 to 1923) described the concept of x-rays. Low-dose x-rays led to mammography as a means to detect breast cancer.

Twentieth Century

- This was the era of epidemiological studies, the introduction of radiotherapy, mammography, and chemotherapy.

Pre-1950

- Geoffrey Keynes (1887 to 1982) treated breast cancer by radium implantation.
- Janet Elizabeth Lane-Claypon (1877 to 1967) published a landmark study on breast cancer risk factors.
- Albert Salomon (1883 to 1976) found microcalcifications in x-ray images of tumor samples, providing substantial information about the pathological differences between cancerous and normal tissues.

- Robert Egan (1920 to 2002) used mammography to diagnose 53 cases of occult breast cancer. He is considered to be the father of modern mammography.

- Robert McWhirter (1904 to 1994) reported the results of a combined use of simple mastectomy followed by radiotherapy in breast cancer treatment.

- Beginning in the 1930s and throughout the decades, there were numerous advances in radiology, including the introduction of radiotherapy as an alternative to radical mastectomy, use of the radium-based interstitial irradiation (brachytherapy), electron beam therapy, and cobalt teletherapy.

Post-1950

- Jacob Gershon-Cohen (1899 to 1971) and Helen Ingleby (1887 to 1973) showed that mammography could help detect breast cancers that could not be discovered on physical examination.

- Bernard Fisher (1918 to 2019) was the first to introduce clinical trials and statistical methodology to breast cancer research. He also showed the effectiveness of lumpectomy, as a means of treating some breast cancers.

- Beginning in the 1970s, radiation therapy to treat cancers included proton beam therapy, stereotactic radiation therapy, adaptive RT (ART), and a special form of image-guided radiotherapy (IGRT).

- In 1966, the first compression mammography machine was developed.

- First Lady Betty Ford (1918 to 2011) was diagnosed with breast cancer. She raised awareness of breast cancer by discussing her disease candidly with the public.

- In 1979, the National Institutes of Health (NIH) concluded that radical mastectomy was no longer an appropriate surgical procedure to treat breast cancer.

- In 1977, tamoxifen was approved to treat advanced breast cancer. In 1986, it was approved as adjuvant therapy for postmenopausal women and in 1998 for prophylactic use in women at high risk of breast cancer.

- In the 1980s, public health advocates encouraged women to perform self-examinations of their breasts and undergo mammography and clinical breast examinations.

- In 1982, Susan G. Komen Breast Cancer Foundation was founded in memory of Susan Komen, who died from breast cancer.

- In 1987, the growth factor receptor gene *HER2*, which produces HER2 proteins, was discovered.

- In 1994, the tumor suppressor genes *BRCA1* and *BRCA2* were identified. The first targeted anti–breast cancer drug, trastuzumab (Herceptin) was approved in combination with paclitaxel chemotherapy in 1998 for HER2-positive metastatic breast cancer. In 2006, Herceptin was also approved as part of adjuvant therapy for women with early-stage HER2-positive breast cancer.

- Research in cancer biology in the 1980s and 1990s led to significant progress in cancer prevention, early detection, and treatment.

Twenty-First Century

- In the 21st century, there was substantial progress in gene and protein expression profiling, targeted therapies, immunotherapy, cancer genetics, nanotechnology, and robotic surgery. There were substantial advances in the molecular classification of breast cancer based on gene expression profiles.

- In 2000, Perou et al. published seminal studies on microarray-based gene expression profiling as a new way of classifying breast cancers.

- In 2003, digital mammography was introduced.

- In 2004, Oncotype DX Breast Cancer Assay enabled a personalized approach to chemotherapy, making it possible to individualize chemotherapy treatments.

- In 2005, the FDA approved a new class of drugs, Aromatase Inhibitors (AIs), which work by lowering estrogen levels. AIs were found to be more effective than tamoxifen in reducing deaths among women with ER-positive breast cancer.

- In 2007, MammaPrint, a 70-genomic test that analyzes the activity of certain genes in early-stage breast cancer, was approved by the FDA. The test can be used to analyze cancers that are hormone-receptor-positive and hormone-receptor-negative. The test also calculates whether the cancer has a low or high risk of recurrence within 10 years after diagnosis.

- In 2007, Raloxifene (EvistaTM) was approved for the prevention of invasive breast cancer in postmenopausal women with osteoporosis and in postmenopausal women at high risk for invasive breast cancer.

- In 2013, Oscar-winning actress Angelina Jolie, who was at high risk of breast cancer because she tested positive for the *BRCA1* gene, publically announced that she had a prophylactic bilateral mastectomy and salpingo-ooprhorectomy.
- Personalized medicine, also called targeted medicine, is made possible by advances in molecular research. On December 18, 2015, President Barack Obama signed the bipartisan Precision Medicine Initiative, defining the effort as "delivering the right treatments, at the right time, every time to the right person."

Source: Adapted from Lukong KE. Understanding breast cancer—The long and winding road. *BBA Clin.* 2017; 7: 64–77.

Treating Breast Cancer in the 21st Century: Is Precision Targeted Cancer Therapy the Wave of the Future?

> It is more important to know what sort of person has a disease than to know what sort of disease a person has.
>
> Hippocrates (460 to 370 BCE)

Cancer *per se* is not one disease. It is a heterogeneous catchall term to denote a malignant growth or tumor resulting from the division of abnormal cells in an uncontrolled way in the body. There are so many pathogenic abnormalities from which a specific cancer might develop, which makes it much more difficult to find a single treatment, much less a cure. Complicating things further, cancer presents in many different forms, depending on the site of the body, and requires an understanding of the underlying molecular abnormalities that drive cancer growth. Treatment for breast cancer, for example, will differ from treatment for brain, lung, or colon cancer.

All cancers are similar in that the malignancy is caused by accumulated damage to genes. There are two main types of genes that play a role in cancer: oncogenes and tumor suppressor genes. An oncogene is a gene that has the potential to cause cancer. Tumor suppressor genes keep the processes of cell growth and cell death (apoptosis) in check, which can serve to suppress tumor development. When a tumor suppressor gene is mutated, this can lead to tumor formation or growth. *BRCA1* and *BRCA2*, for example, are tumor suppressor genes. While having a *BRCA1* and *BRCA2* gene mutation raises the risk of developing cancer, there is not a 100% guarantee that cancer will develop. Exposure to cancer-causing substances such as chemicals, radiation, tobacco smoke, or inherited gene defects also could predispose an individual to developing cancer. Emphasis should be placed on "could," as individuals may have the same exposure to potentially cancer-causing factors, but not everyone will actually develop cancer. It is complicated!

There is now a much better understanding of the series of genetic changes that trigger cells to malfunction, causing cells to grow uncontrollably into malignant tumors. Of course, there is still much to learn about the mysteries of cancer, but knowledge about the genetic basis of cancer today is far superior to that of just a decade or so ago. While much is made of an inherited susceptibility of breast cancer, in actuality most breast cancers arise from genetic changes that occur over a lifetime. My mother, for example, was the only female in her family to develop breast cancer, and so far neither her sister, my sisters, nor I have been diagnosed with breast cancer. When she was first diagnosed several decades ago, harnessing the power of molecular markers for breast cancer was still in its infancy. Since that time, there has been tremendous advancement in molecular biology, unfortunately a bit too late to benefit my mother and others like her.

The Promise of Cancer Biology

There is no doubt that research in cancer biology during the past 40 years, especially within the past 20 years, has led to substantial progress in cancer detection, treatment, and prevention. In particular, there has been dramatic progress in gene and protein expression profiling, immunotherapy, nanotechnology, and cancer genetics. For many cancer treatments, reliance on a toxic, systematic course of chemotherapy has yielded to a more efficient, target-directed therapy. And over the past five years, there have been substantial advances in the molecular subclassification of many cancers, leading to the development of targeted treatments that permit the customization of cancer treatment. Targeted therapy is a much more precise approach, taking into account the unique situation in one patient, rather than generalizing treatment to fit all patients. Indeed, one of the most promising and exciting areas within personalized medicine is the field of pharmacogenetics, which focuses on how an individual's genetic makeup influences treatment effectiveness. One size does not necessarily fit all when it comes to cancer treatment.

Identifying genetic biomarkers is key to targeted therapies. With breast cancer, for example, targeted therapy takes into account the presence or absence of receptors for estrogen, progesterone, and the *HER2* gene. With this knowledge, specific treatment can be tailored to the individual. Today, for example, women with hormone receptor positive tumors typically are prescribed a selective estrogen-receptor response modulator (SERM) drug and/or an aromatase inhibitor (AI), while those with HER-2/neu overexpressing tumors typically receive anti-HER2 targeted therapy in combination with chemotherapy (i.e., extra *HER2* genes cause breast cells to make too many HER2 receptors—HER2 protein overexpression—that make breast cells grow and divide in an uncontrolled way).[1] The widely prescribed drug, Herceptin, discussed in the previous chapter, is a novel HER2 targeting agent. Those with triple-negative breast cancer, especially those with the *BRCA* mutation, unfortunately still have more limited treatment options (usually a combination of chemotherapeutic drugs are given). On a more positive note, new, emerging biological and immunological therapies are now available, and there are many more in the research pipeline that are designed to specifically target molecular subtypes of breast and other cancers, which hopefully will improve prognosis for survival.

Since cancer is caused by certain changes to genes that control the way cells function, especially how they grow and divide, research has focused on the molecular level in hopes of understanding better the mysteries of cancer development. For more than one decade, over 1,000 scientists in 37 countries have collaboratively worked to analyze the whole genetic code of 2,658 cancers.[2] Their work, published in 2020 in the journal *Nature*, provides a wealth of information that inevitably will help unlock the secrets of cancer development and ultimately lead to treatment modalities that can be tailored to an individual's unique tumor. The project found that cancer as a whole is very complex (but we already knew that!), as thousands of different combinations of mutations are responsible for the development of a malignancy.

On average, cancers contain fundamental mutations that could precipitate a cancer's growth by accelerating unchecked cell division rates that could lead to a malignancy. This being the case, and with this knowledge, diagnosis and treatment of these "driver mutations" are more possible now than ever before. Cancer biologists focus on the mechanisms of cell growth, the transformation of normal cells to cancer cells, and the spread (metastasis) of cancer cells. The big challenge is to develop diagnostic tests that can differentiate mutations that would become cancer from those that probably would not and to differentiate what is normal from what is not.

Another challenge is to better understand drug resistance, a major factor in the failure of many forms of chemotherapy. Basically, this means that the cancer cells resist the effects of the chemotherapy. While we may not fully understand the reasons for drug resistance, we do know that cancer has the ability to become resistant to many different types of drugs. There are many plausible explanations for this, including the possibility that there may be more resistant cells than cells that are sensitive to the chemotherapy, or the protein that transports the drug across the cell wall stops working. Currently, 90% of failures in patients undergoing chemotherapy are related to drug resistance.[3] Research in cancer genomics is helping to understand the major components that contribute the drug resistance. But because of the heterogeneity in mutations in multiple and different cancer-causing genes, personalized therapies are required. For this reason, among others, targeted cancer therapy, sometimes called precision medicine, is viewed by those in the medical profession as having so much potential.

What Is Precision/Personalized Medicine?

Precision medicine, also in the past referred to as personalized medicine, focuses on finding the "best" treatment most likely to help an individual patient, taking into account their genetic, environmental, and lifestyle factors. Precision medicine does not mean that treatment is unique to an individual *per se*; rather, based on genetic knowledge, individuals can be classified into subgroups with similar genetic characteristics. That is, individuals with similar molecular profiles would benefit from a specific treatment, whereas those without that profile probably would not. Although "personalized medicine" seems to imply this meaning, the thinking was that the term could be misinterpreted as implying that unique treatments can be designed for each individual, which is not exactly the case.[4] The term "personalized medicine" is generally not used now; rather, "precision medicine" is viewed as better reflecting the scope and purpose of this new approach for treating diseases.

In January 2015, President Obama announced in his State of the Union address the Precision Medicine Initiative, which was intended "to accelerate a new era of medicine that delivers the right treatment at the right time to the right person, taking into account individuals' health history, genes, environments, and lifestyles."[5] On December 18, 2015, the president signed bipartisan legislation providing $215 million for the Precision Medicine Initiative. One of the key initiatives focused on cancer treatment. The National Cancer Institute (NCI) was allocated $70 million to fund research to identify genomic drivers in cancer and apply that knowledge in the development of more effective approaches to cancer treatment, including funding to expand genetically based clinical cancer trials, explore fundamental aspects of cancer biology, and establish a national cancer knowledge network designed to generate and share knowledge to guide treatment decisions.

In order to fully realize the goals of the Precision Medicine Initiative, a genomic database is needed to be developed. By way of explanation, the genome is an organism's complete set of its hereditary information encoded in its DNA (or, for some viruses, RNA). In humans, for example, the genome is the set of genetic information encoded in 46 chromosomes found in the nucleus of each cell. Genomic databases allow for the storing, sharing, and comparison of data across research studies, across data types, across individuals, and across organisms. Today, there are thousands of genomic databases, tools, and other resources freely accessible on the Internet.[6] The Human Genome Project is one such example.

One of the primary goals of the Human Genome Project is to provide a complete and accurate sequence of the 3 billion DNA base pairs that make up the human genome and to find all of the estimated 20,000 to 25,000 human genes. Beginning on October 1, 1990, and completed in April 2003, the Human Genome Project provided, for the first time, the ability to produce the complete genetic blueprint, which enables scientists to develop highly effective diagnostic tools to better understand the health needs of people based on their individual genetic makeup and to design new and highly effective treatments for disease. This was an ambitious project indeed, but one that certainly helped to advance medical science.[7]

One novel invention developed within the past two decades, microarray technology, has important applications in pharmacogenomics, drug discovery and development, drug safety, and molecular diagnostics. For example, DNA biochip microarray is a tool used to determine whether the DNA from a particular individual contains a mutation in genes. Biochip microarrays are a collection of small glass slides (microarrays) holding up to hundreds of thousands of tiny spots of DNA, each targeted to a specific gene. Biochips are essentially miniaturized laboratories that can perform hundreds or thousands of simultaneous biochemical reactions. Gene expression profiling by microarrays is helping the progress of personalized cancer treatment based on the molecular classification of subtypes.[8]

In summary, while physicians have always tried to tailor a therapy or treatment to best fit the needs of the patient, in many instances important information about the patient (i.e., genetic information) was not available, thus essentially limiting the ability to tailor the treatment with high precision. For example, not so long ago therapy and treatments for breast cancer were limited in that the molecular and genetic signature of the patient was not known. Thus, administering a specific chemotherapy for all breast cancer patients would work for some but not for all, given the differences in the specific molecular composition of the cancer. By understanding the molecular targets of the cancer (i.e., *BRCA1* or *BRCA2* mutation or HER2-positive or negative breast cancer), therapy can be much more targeted and precise. Precision medicine relies on genomic data to make decisions about which treatment should be prescribed. It can identify protein markers of a disease before clinical presentation. It can be used in decision-making about preemptive interventions. Precision medicine has the potential to revolutionize how we treat disease in a much more targeted, efficient way.

What Is Targeted Cancer Therapy?

In contrast to chemotherapy, which interferes with cell division and kills the rapidly dividing normal and cancerous cells, targeted cancer therapy is intended to block tumor cell proliferation. Targeted cancer therapy (sometimes also referred to as molecularly targeted drugs, molecularly targeted therapies, or precision medicine) relies on anticancer drugs to block the growth and/or spread of cancer by interfering with specific molecules (i.e., molecular targets) that are involved in the growth, progression, and spread of the cancer.[9] That is, targeted cancer therapy works by targeting the cancer's specific genes, proteins, or the tissue environment that contributes to cancer growth. Since understanding an individual's genetic profile and the type of proteins in the cancer cells is imperative in targeted cancer therapy, prior to initiating a targeted therapy, tests would be done to compare the amount of individual proteins in cancer cells with those in normal cells.

Protein targeting is an important component of targeted therapy. Not all tumors have the same targets, and the same targeted treatment will not necessarily work for everyone. Determining whether, or which, cancer cells produce mutant (altered) proteins that drive cancer progression is the key to unlock the ability of a therapy to work effectively. Targeting fusion genes (i.e., a gene that incorporates parts of two different genes whose product is called a fusion protein) is another means of targeted therapy. Knowing the type of proteins that are present in cancer cells or specific types of proteins that are found to be more abundant in cancer cells than in normal cells would be very helpful so as to determine if the specific targeted therapy would be effective, and, if so, to what extent. Clearly, testing the tumor's genes or other molecular features can help doctors decide which treatments may be best for an individual with cancer, regardless of where the cancer is located or how it looks under the microscope.[10]

Although most current cancer treatments treat the malignant tumor that developed in a specific organ or tissue (i.e., breast, lung, colon), there are therapies being used to treat any kind of cancer as long as the cancer has the specific molecular alteration targeted by the drug. Such therapies focus on tumor agonists and antagonists. A tumor agonist is a substance that acts like another substance and stimulates an action to produce a biological response. Whereas an agonist causes an action, an antagonist blocks the action of the agonist. Agonist and antagonist immunotherapy, for example, has become a powerful clinical strategy for treating cancer by using the immune system to attack cancer cells through natural mechanisms with the aim of creating antitumor immune responses.[11]

Exciting research is being conducted in the area of cancer immunotherapy. Immunotherapies are a form of biotherapy (also called biologic therapy or biological response modifier [BRM] therapy) because they use materials from living organisms to fight disease.[12] Essentially this type of therapy works by turning one's immune system against the tumor, but interactions between tumor cells and the immune system are complex, and in some instances, the therapy can cause the immune system to attack cancer cells as well as healthy cells.[13] This is still a young science, and much more research needs to be conducted to enable oncologists to understand which patients are the best candidates for immunotherapies and which immunotherapies work best on specific cancers.

Without getting too deep into the weeds, suffice it to say that immunotherapy focuses on ways a type of cancer treatment can be used to boost the body's natural defenses to fight cancer cells. As of this writing, immunotherapy is not yet appropriate for all cancers, but is being used in the treatment of some melanoma; bladder, kidney, head, and neck cancers; non-Hodgkin's lymphoma; and non-small-cell lung cancer.

Research in immunology is also focusing on monoclonal antibodies as a means of therapy. The immune system attacks foreign substances by making large numbers of antibodies, proteins that stick to a specific protein called an antigen. Antigens are identified by the immune systems as being harmful to the body. Antibodies are naturally produced in the immune system to specifically target a certain antigen, such as one found on cancer cells. Additionally, it is possible to create antibodies in the laboratory.

Monoclonal antibodies, defined as an antibody produced by a single clone of cells or cell line and consisting of identical antibody molecules, are designed to bind with an antigen to empower the body's immune system to target and destroy the cells containing the antigen. Stated another way, monoclonal antibodies are laboratory-produced molecules engineered to serve as substitute antibodies that can restore, enhance, or mimic the immune system's attack on cancer cells.[14] Each type of monoclonal antibody will target a specific targeted antigen in the body.

Monoclonal antibodies work in different ways, depending on the antigen they are targeting. For example, some monoclonal antibodies mark cancer cells so that the immune system will better recognize and destroy them. Some monoclonal antibody drugs block protein-cell interactions necessary for the development of new blood vessels. This is important, as cancer can spread to other parts of the body through the bloodstream or lymphatic system where new tumors can grow (i.e., circulating tumor cells). Bevacizumab (sold under the trade name Avastin[R]), for example, prevents tumors from making new blood vessels that could feed the tumor, essentially cutting off the cancer cells from all nutrients. Cancer cells need blood to grow and proliferate.

While the immunology of monoclonal antibodies may sound confusing to the layperson, it is easy to identify them! The name of the drug gives a clue. Monoclonal antibodies end with the stem "-mab." For example, trastuzumab (Herceptin) and ipilimumab (Yervoy) are monoclonal antibodies used in cancer treatment.[15] Monoclonal antibodies can be used for many purposes other than fighting cancer, including testing for pregnancy by detecting HCG hormones in urine and testing for diseases such herpes, chlamydia, and HIV.

There also are antibodies that work by blocking pathways that are critical to the immune system's ability to control cancer growth. These pathways are called immune checkpoints, and the specific antibodies are referred to as immune checkpoint inhibitors, which work by having immune cells (i.e., T cells) recognize and attack tumors. Nonspecific immunotherapies such as interferons and interleukins also help the immune system to destroy cancer cells or slow the growth of the cancer. Many immunotherapy treatments are used in combination with surgery, chemotherapy, radiation, or targeted therapies to improve their effectiveness.

Other cancer immunotherapies include vaccines and T cell infusions. A medical definition from MedicineNet, worded for the layperson, explains that T cells are like soldiers who search out and destroy the targeted invaders.[16] There is ongoing research focusing on producing T cells that can more effectively target cancer and other hard-to-treat diseases that can evade the normal immune system. Without going into the complexities of immunology of T cells, suffice it to say that they have an important role within the immune system.

There are many other types of targeted therapy used in cancer treatment, including hormone therapies (talked about in the previous chapter), signal transduction inhibitors, gene expression modulators, apoptosis (controlled cell death) inducers, angiogenesis inhibitors (blocking the growth of new blood vessels to tumors), and toxin delivery molecules. Hormone therapies, for example, are being used in breast and prostate cancer treatments and act by preventing the body from producing the hormones or by interfering with the action of the hormones.

Another component that needs to be discussed is the importance of pharmacogenetics, the branch of pharmacology focused on the effect of genetic factors on reactions to drugs—that is, to what extent will an individual respond to a specific pharmaceutical intervention based on his or her unique genetic makeup. It is now possible for physicians to order a genetic test to ascertain to what extent the individual would benefit, or not, from a specific drug treatment. To what extent would an individual's genetic makeup reduce the effectiveness of the drug treatment?

But There Are Limitations

Unfortunately, there are limitations to the application of the various forms of targeted cancer therapy discussed in previous chapters. Not every cancer patient will be a candidate for targeted therapy. In order for targeted therapy to "work," the cancerous tumor must have a specific gene mutation that codes for the target. Patients who do not have the mutation would not be a candidate for targeted cancer therapy because the therapy would have nothing to target. Furthermore, there are instances when the cancer cells become resistant to the therapy. That is, the tumor finds a new pathway to achieve tumor growth that does not depend on the target; thus, the targeted therapy would become irrelevant. One way to address this situation is to combine the targeted therapy with another type of treatment (i.e., chemotherapy). Further, targeted cancer therapy has side effects, including gastrointestinal problems; skin problems (acneiform rash, dry skin, nail changes, hair depigmentation); and problems with blood clotting, wound healing, and high blood pressure.[17]

While advances in immunotherapy are exciting and offer hope for a cancer cure, in reality relatively few cancer patients actually benefit from the treatment. At this point in time, researchers estimate that for two-thirds (68.8%) of cancers there are no immunotherapy options.[18] That being said, in early 2020, a new type of immune T cell was discovered by accident by British scientists, a finding that could usher in a major breakthrough in cancer treatment. The researchers said that their finding raises the prospect of a "one-size-fits-all" cancer treatment, a single type of T cell that could be capable of destroying many different types of cancers across the population, laying the foundation for a "universal" T cell medicine.[19] Of course, much more needs to be done to assess how this new T cell works before we let ourselves get too excited.

The FDA has approved numerous targeted therapies for many different cancers, and there are ongoing clinical trials that are testing types of targeted therapies. The National Cancer Institute (NCI) has a helpful website that lists NCI-supported clinical trials (https://www.cancer.gov/about-cancer/treatment /clinical-trials/search).

Is It All Science Fiction?

Advances in genomic profiling and testing are progressing at a rapid pace, enabling oncologists to understand the genetic information related to an individual or specific cell type as well as the way their genes interact with each other and with the environment. Genome-wide profiling technologies have enabled a clearer understanding of the biological heterogeneity of breast cancer. Understanding distinct gene signatures has led to novel therapeutic approaches. The 21-gene Recurrence Score (RS) assay (Oncotype DX® Breast Recurrence Score assay, Genomic Health Inc.), for example, is a tumor profiling test that makes it possible to individualize treatments by analyzing the expression patterns (i.e., signature) of 21 genes in breast tumor tissues. The assay can help predict outcomes for patients by determining the likelihood that chemotherapy would be beneficial and is now used widely to guide treatment decisions in estrogen receptor (ER)–positive and human epidermal growth factor receptor 2 (HER2)–negative node-negative breast cancer.[20]

Genomic profiling and testing is highly sophisticated and can provide highly technical data to the oncologist. What about DNA testing kits that are sold to the consumer? A growing number of companies are marketing genetic testing kits directly to consumers, many of which are sold directly to consumers on the Internet. Probably the best known of these type of tests are AncestryDNA as well as 23andMe. How accurate and effective are they?

The axiom "Buyer beware" is an apt analogy, as many of these kits have been found to be inaccurate and interpretation of the results may be misleading to the consumer. I bring up the issue of genetic testing kits because someone might want to know how effective they are. In no way should these tests be considered to be at the same level of the tests discussed earlier. There is no comparison! These types of testing cannot tell definitively whether you will or will not get a particular disease. Further, the results of genetic testing may affect your ability to obtain life, disability, or long-term care insurance.

The direct-to-consumer genetic testing kits are not used in targeted/personalized medicine. They should never be considered to be anything more than raising awareness of a potential disease or disorder, which should be assessed and tested by your physician in a more sophisticated way. And a geneticist or genetic counselor should first be consulted to discuss the pros and cons of genetic testing as well as the possible social and emotional aspects of testing. These professionals will help interpret the results of the testing and collaborate with your physician. It is one thing to take a pregnancy test in the privacy of your home. It is another to take a genetic test without appropriate professional input.

Wouldn't it be wonderful if there was a tool to "fix"/edit genes? The CRISPR (clustered regular interspaced short palindromic repeats) system uses gene editing to alter DNA sequences and modify gene function. This could enable scientists to repair genetic defects or use genetically modified human cells as therapies. In fact, scientists at Boston Children's Hospital and Northeastern University have developed a CRISPR genome editing system that suppresses the growth of triple-negative breast cancer, the most deadly form of breast cancer.[21] While still in its experimental phase, CRISPR genome editing shows promise as a potential treatment or even cure for genetic diseases including cancer.

Other similar prognostic decision tools have been developed not only for breast cancer but also for other cancers such as lung and ovarian, enabling oncologists to make decisions about the value of specific therapies for a specific patient based on his or her tumor type. While this used to be the fodder for science fiction, today it is no longer a pipedream. It is reality.

CHAPTER TEN

Complementary, Alternative, and Integrated Medicine

While the preceding chapters discussed current treatment options for breast cancer patients, this chapter will explore complementary, alternative, and integrated medicine (CAM) options and therapies that individuals could considered using *in conjunction with* conventional therapies. CAM therapies should not be viewed as a substitute or replacement for conventional treatments; rather, they can be used along with conventional treatments.

What Is Complementary, Alternative, and Integrated Medicine?

The National Cancer Institute (NCI) categorizes complementary and alternative therapies as medical products and practices that are not part of standard medical care. *Complementary medicine* refers to treatments that are not considered to be standard or conventional treatments, but they can be used along with such medical treatments (i.e., acupuncture to help lessen side effects of cancer treatment). *Alternative medicine* refers to treatments that are used instead of standard medical treatments (i.e., a special diet to treat cancer instead of anticancer drugs). Integrative medicine is defined as a healing-oriented medicine that addresses the full range of physical, emotional, mental, social, spiritual, and environmental influences that affect a person's health. The Integrated medicine's approach is to utilize effective treatments from different disciplines, including conventional medicine and complementary therapies, to treat the whole patient. Practitioners of integrated medicine utilize holistic healing modalities in addition to conventional treatments in their practice. Practitioners of holistic health address the physical, emotional, social, spiritual, and physical health of an individual. That is, holistic health takes into account the whole person, body, mind, and spirit, in the quest for optimal health and wellness, which may include diet, exercise, psychotherapy, and relationship and spiritual counseling.

In many respects, there is overlap in definition and purpose of complementary, alternative, and integrated medicine. However, integrated medicine is a medical specialty just like medicine or pediatrics, and doctors can become board certified in integrative medicine just as they do in medicine or pediatrics. This is not the case with complementary or alternative medicine. There also is a subspecialty in integrated oncology, which, as the name implies, focuses on treating cancer patients using the principles of integrated medicine. In order to keep things simple, I will use CAM as the catchall phrase to embody complementary, alternative, and integrated medicine.

As the diagram shows, CAM is divided into five major domains: Whole Medical Systems, Mind-Body Interventions, Manipulative and Body-Based Practices, Energy Medicine, and Biological-Based Practices.[1]

Whole Medical Systems refer to traditional Chinese medicine (i.e., acupuncture), Ayurveda (i.e., holistic healing), naturopathy (i.e., herbs, massage, acupuncture, exercise, and nutritional counseling), and homeopathy (i.e., use of plants and minerals in diluted forms to stimulate the healing process).

Mind-Body Interventions focus on the relationships between the mind, body, spirit, and behavior, and the belief is that the mind can regulate bodily functions and symptoms. Examples include meditation, breathing, yoga, hypnosis, biofeedback, tai chi, and visual imagery. Music therapy is also included in this domain.

Manipulative and Body-Based Practices include traditional Chinese medicine, homeopathy, naturopathy; Ayurveda, acupuncture, massage therapy, hypnosis, meditation, biofeedback, yoga, and tai chi. Also included is chiropractic and osteopathic manipulation.

Energy Medicine (sometimes referred to as energy healing or spiritual healing) is a traditional healing system that restores the balance and flow of energy throughout the body, mind, and soul and is used often to treat ailments related to mental health. The objective is to restore homeostasis in the organism. Examples include the use of electromagnetic therapy, Reiki, and Qigong.

Biological-Based Practices include use of herbs, dietary supplements, and probiotics. Unlike pharmaceutical products, biology-based supplements are not subject to rigorous testing to prove their safety and effectiveness for treatment. Natural does not necessarily mean safe. Therefore, the efficacy of many biology-based substances remains unsubstantiated.

CAM is used in the treatment of a wide variety of medical conditions. The use of CAM therapies in cancer care, however, tend to focus on reduction of anxiety/stress; alleviation of mood disorders (i.e., sadness, depression);

improvement in quality of life and physical functioning; and mitigation of chemotherapy-induced nausea and vomiting, pain, sleep disturbance, and fatigue. Of course, there are many pharmaceutical options to address these side effects of cancer care, but many women are asking that CAM therapies be included in the treatment regime as a means to manage treatment-related side effects.

The big question is how safe and how effective are CAM therapies? What are the potential benefits and potential harms of CAM therapies? Importantly, to what extent will a CAM therapy interact in a negative/harmful way with conventional treatment? The purpose of using CAM therapies is not to place the patient in danger by causing serious adverse events that might occur during conventional treatment.

There are skeptics of CAM therapies who question the value and safety of some CAM therapies. A large part of the problem is that the efficacy and effectiveness of some CAM treatments are poorly understood. Complicating the issue is that it is difficult to assess the efficacy and safety of CAM therapies in rigorous clinical trials, the cornerstone of mainstream cancer care. That being said, a majority of cancer patients will use some CAM therapies during treatment in addition to conventional treatments, but they should do so with the full knowledge and support of their physician. While some CAM therapies are benign (i.e., yoga, meditation, massage), others are more invasive (i.e., acupuncture) or possibly dangerous because they could interact in a harmful way with conventional treatments (i.e., dietary supplements, herbal supplements). No cancer patient should take it upon herself to self-treat with CAM without her doctor's knowledge and permission.

Some CAM therapies have undergone careful evaluation and have been found to be safe and effective. However, there are others that could be ineffective or possibly harmful (i.e., some botanicals and nutritional products, including dietary supplements, herbal supplements, and vitamins). Just as standard cancer treatments need to be rigorously studied in clinical trials for safety and effectiveness, CAM therapies also need to be evaluated to assess safety, efficacy, and effectiveness.

CAM Oversight

The National Center for Complementary and Integrative Health (NCCIH), formerly known as the National Center for Complementary and Alternative Medicine, is part of the National Institutes of Health (NIH) that is responsible for scientific research on complementary and integrative health approaches. Its mission is to quantify, through rigorous scientific investigation, the usefulness and safety of complementary and integrative health interventions and the extent to which such therapies improve health and well-being.[2]

Further, the NCI's Office of Cancer Complementary and Alternative Medicine (OCCAM) was established to coordinate activities of the NCI in CAM research as it relates to the prevention, diagnosis, and treatment of cancer, cancer-related symptoms, and side effects of conventional cancer treatment.[3]

The NCI and the NCCIH fund clinical trials designed to assess CAM treatments and therapies. Examples of such trials include a study to assess the effectiveness of acupuncture to help improve the cognitive difficulties and insomnia that many cancer survivors report following chemotherapy and other cancer treatments; a trial looking at auricular point acupressure as a means to help reduce the side effects of aromatase inhibitor treatment; and a study designed to evaluate an intensive meditation-based stress reduction intervention's efficacy in improving cognitive functioning among breast cancer survivors.[4]

What Does the Evidence Show?

Anxiety, stress, fatigue, and mood disturbances are common among cancer patients. Of course, there are pharmaceutical drugs that could be prescribed to address these symptoms, but there are also other means to help alleviate the feelings of anxiety and stress as well as sadness and depression so as to enhance quality of life. In particular, cancer-related fatigue, including feeling weak, worn-out, sluggish, and having no energy, is much more than just feeling tired. Fatigue can have a negative impact on one's quality of life, mood, and self-esteem and should not be ignored by the patient and health care team.

Pain is a known by-product of cancer treatment, and pain management needs to be managed by trained clinicians. It requires proper assessment, as each individual experiences pain differently. Pain can negatively impact one's physical and mental state and should be treated rather than ignored. Evidence shows that there are no CAM therapies recommended to alleviate pain, although used in conjunction with pharmacological treatments some CAM therapies can help.

There are conditions that present during and after cancer treatment for which there are no reliably good CAM therapies. For example, radiation dermatitis is a common side effect in breast cancer patients for which there are limited effective CAM therapies. There are no effective CAM therapies for hot flashes or lymphedema, common side effects of breast cancer treatment. Cancer treatment may cause damage to the peripheral nerves (chemotherapy-induced peripheral neuropathy), but there are no recommended CAM therapies for this condition. Even though sleep disturbances are common among those undergoing cancer treatment, there are no CAM therapies that are recommended to improve sleep quality.

The literature on CAM studies highlights the difficulty in designing and conducting a well-designed study to assess safety, efficacy, and effectiveness of CAM therapies. How does one conduct a randomized placebo-controlled trial on therapies that are difficult to quantify in the first place? Fatigue, pain, and moods, for example, are highly subjective, and trying to quantify improvement using a CAM therapy can be difficult.

A 2017 clinical practice guideline issued by the Society for Integrative Oncology (Society) focuses on the use of a wide range of CAM therapies during and after breast cancer treatment.[5] The researchers conducted a systematic review of the literature from 1990 to 2015 and focused only on randomized clinical trials, the gold standard used in clinical research to assess the safety, efficacy, and effectiveness of pharmaceutical drugs and medical devices. The guidelines, based on the best evidence in the published literature, do not address breast cancer recurrence or survival primarily because there are no trials looking at the effect of CAM therapies on these outcomes.

The focus and purpose of the guidelines is an assessment of the effectiveness of CAM therapies on managing symptoms as well as quantifying side effects (serious or benign) during and after breast cancer treatment. While there are scores of CAM therapies available, the following presents a listing of only those that the Society recommends based on the strength of the evidence, taking into account quality of the trial, sample size, consistency of results among trials, and statistical significance. The Society graded each therapy based on the available evidence: the therapy is recommended (i.e., there is high certainty that the net benefit is substantial or that there is moderate certainty that the net benefit is moderate to substantial); the evidence of effectiveness is equivocal; the net benefit is small; and the evidence did not show any benefit (therapies that fall into this category will not be presented here). It is important to stress that the CAM therapies listed here are not stand-alone therapies; rather, they are used in conjunction with standard therapy and can be combined (i.e., more than one CAM therapy can be used at the same time).

Acupuncture: Acupuncture is used to alleviate chemotherapy-induced nausea and vomiting, pain management, hot flashes, fatigue, stress, anxiety, and sleep disorders. Studies show that breast cancer patients undergoing chemotherapy benefit from acupuncture, which should be done along with standard care for nausea and vomiting. It is important that the therapy is done by a trained, licensed acupuncturist.

Acupressure: Acupressure is used to alleviate pain, fatigue, and stress. A trained therapist applies pressure to specific points on the body (acupoints).

Ayurvedic Medicine (Ayurveda): Developed over 3,000 years ago in India, Ayurveda is one of the world's oldest holistic natural healing system. Among the components of Ayurveda are diet, exercise, meditation, yoga, herbs, massage, and controlled breathing.

Cognitive Behavioral Stress Management: Patients are taught coping skills to reduce stress and to relax. A cognitive behavioral therapist should oversee this therapy.

Dietary Supplements: There are thousands of dietary supplements available to the consumer. In the United States, the law defines dietary supplements, available over-the-counter without a prescription, as products taken by mouth that contain a "dietary ingredient" (i.e., vitamins, minerals, botanicals, herbs, amino acids, enzyme supplements, and herbs or botanicals). These products are not regulated by the Federal Drug Administration (FDA), and there is no standardization of such products, although dietary supplement firms must report to the FDA any serious adverse events that are reported to them by consumers or health care professionals. How many actually do so is subject to debate. Further, the manufacturer or seller does not have to prove to FDA's satisfaction that the claim listed on the label is accurate or truthful before it appears on the product. Buyers, beware. You may not know what you are ingesting.

Some common dietary supplements used by cancer patients include *ginger*, which is used for chemotherapy-induced nausea and vomiting; however, it should not be taken by individuals with bleeding disorders. *Ginseng* is used to treat cancer-related fatigue; however, there are potentially serious side effects of taking ginseng, including headaches, rapid heart rate, low blood sugar, and gastrointestinal problems. *Antioxidants* such as vitamins C, A, and E as well as coenzyme Q10 and carotenoids are taken to boost the immune system, but may increase the risk of breast cancer recurrence. CBD supplements may be taken to relieve pain, but the evidence of pain relief in people with cancer is scarce.

Cancer patients, in particular, must exercise caution when making a decision to take dietary supplements. Some supplements may cause serious complications (i.e., curcumin has tumor-inhibiting action, but interacts with anticoagulant drugs). Anyone considering adding dietary supplements for their treatment should seek their physician's advice about which supplements can be safely taken with chemotherapy or other cancer treatments. What are the potential side effects/harms/interactions of the supplement with chemotherapy or other cancer treatments? What does the evidence show about the effectiveness of the supplement?

Hypnosis: Hypnosis is used for relaxation and to help relieve stress, anxiety, and pain. An individual trained in hypnosis should oversee this therapy.

Massage: The goal of massage is to promote relaxation and alleviate muscle stiffness and pain. Massage therapy also can help improve mood and overall quality of life. A trained massage therapist should be used and care must be taken not to massage vulnerable areas of the body (i.e., tumor site, chemo ports, sensitive skin postradiation therapy) too hard. There are many different forms of massage, and the trained therapist will select the best one for the individual.

Mindfulness Meditation: Mindfulness meditation is used to promote calmness and general mental well-being. Mindfulness-Based Stress Reduction (MBSR) is used commonly in cancer care. MBSR is an eight-week program designed to focus on mindfulness in day-to-day life. The evidence shows that mindfulness meditation (group or solo) is effective in reducing anxiety and stress as well as depression. Studies have shown that meditation in general can improve one's quality of life. Meditation has almost no risk to the individual. Is mindfulness meditation "better" than individual counseling? It depends on the individual. There are no studies that compare mindfulness meditation with other similar types of interventions.

Music Therapy: The exact mechanism by which music therapy works is not well understood, but there is evidence that it can provide a calming effect on patients. Qualified music therapists work with the patient to select the "best" interventions (i.e., listening to music, patient producing live music or song). Evidence shows that music therapy can help reduce anxiety and stress. There are no risks to the individuals who engage in music therapy.

Relaxation Techniques: The NCI defines relaxation techniques as including progressive muscle relaxation, biofeedback, self-hypnosis, guided imagery (i.e., patient focuses on pleasant imagery to replace negative or stressful feelings), autogenic training (i.e., concentrating on physical sensations of warmth, heaviness, and relaxation in different parts of the body), and deep breathing exercises. Relaxation therapy has been shown to improve mood. Often, relaxation techniques are combined with other stress management interventions such as guided imagery. Relaxation therapy is noninvasive and risk-free.

Qigong: This form of traditional Chinese medicine integrates movement, meditation, and controlled breathing. "qi" refers to life force or vital energy that flows through the body. In cancer care, qigong is used to reduce anxiety, fatigue, and pain.

Yoga: This mind-body technique, of which there are numerous types, is used for a variety of conditions, including reduction in stress, anxiety, and mood. Yoga is recommended for reducing anxiety and stress, and studies have shown short-term positive effects of yoga on improved quality of life and psychological health. Yoga is noninvasive and essentially risk-free; however, initially one should be guided by a certified yoga instructor to minimize any potential harm such as strained muscles and sprains.

Are CAMs Commonly Used?

It is almost impossible to get an accurate accounting of the use of CAM therapies in general and for cancer care in particular. The first nationally representative survey of prevalence, costs, and patterns of use of CAM was conducted by telephone in 1990. Of the random sample of 1,539 adults who responded, one-third said that they had used at least one type of CAM therapy during the past year to treat their most serious or bothersome medical condition(s).[6] Since that time, that figure has doubled, although it is difficult to get a precise estimate of how many Americans actually use one or more CAM therapies and how frequently.

Multiple studies have found that within one year, up to 80% of patients with cancer used at least one type of CAM therapy during or after treatment.[7,8] Many cancer patients try one or more CAM therapies as a means to moderate side effects of chemotherapy or radiation. Others believe that use of CAM therapies can provide other benefits such as promoting health, managing disease symptoms, preventing illness, or improving immune function.[9] In general, women tend to use CAM therapies more than men.

Concluding Thoughts

Receiving a diagnosis of cancer is a life-changing moment, and most cancer patients will want to try even unproven therapies to obtain a cure. This is understandable. However, a potentially serious issue is that oftentimes the provider will not discuss CAM options with the patient, and the patient will not bring up the issue for fear that their doctor will disapprove. It is possible that some patients do not let their doctor know that they are using CAM unless specifically asked by their health care team. In fact, studies suggest that about 60% of patients who use CAM therapy do not disclose that use to their primary care provider.[10] Not disclosing this information could jeopardize the effectiveness of conventional therapy or even cause potentially serious adverse reactions. While many CAM therapies are benign (i.e., relaxation techniques, meditation, yoga), others can possible cause harm (i.e., some dietary and herbal supplements).

Today, many cancer centers are including integrated medicine/CAM therapies into their cancer program. This allows the patient and the medical team to discuss options and choose the "best" CAM therapies to help the patient deal with the ordeal of her cancer treatment *in a safe manner*. Use of CAM therapies has the potential to help improve quality of life, but what may work for one individual may not for another. The impact of these therapies is highly individualized. Patients and providers need to communicate with each other and form a partnership throughout the course of treatment, and if the patient wants to use CAM therapies, she should be able to do so *with the approval* from her physician and should be monitored for complications as they may arise.

CHAPTER ELEVEN

Coping with Breast Cancer

A diagnosis of any cancer signifies an uncertain future filled with medical procedures, tests, and treatments, each with its own set of side effects and unknowns. Being diagnosed with breast cancer brings forth a complex set of issues that the individual must confront: changes in the physical being, handling the myriad of psychological reactions to the news, concern for the family, wondering how one's loved ones will cope with their wife/mother/daughter/aunt/grandmother's disease, and facing the existential issues of life and death and what it will mean to live life as a cancer patient/survivor.[1] Many breast cancer patients being treated for their disease describe themselves as being on an emotional roller coaster. The ups and downs of treatment, hopes dashed as one treatment fails and another tried, can test the most stalwart.

Although there have been tremendous advances in cancer research that have led to increased survival, the emotional upheavals that a diagnosis of breast cancer unleashes are not insignificant. For many women, it is a time of realization that one's life will never be the same as before a cancer diagnosis. There is an acute awareness of one's vulnerability and mortality. Being told that one has cancer unleashes a cascade of emotions: denial, disbelief, fear of death, anger, grief, vulnerability, anxiety, and, in some cases, depression. There is a feeling of loss of control over one's life.

The disfiguring treatments of surgery and the toxic effects of chemotherapy and radiation individually and collectively have psychological ramifications. Breast cancer, which usually necessitates the removal of all or some of the breast, presents different psychological challenges compared to colon or ovarian cancer, for example, the results of which are out of sight. While surgery will leave a scar that in time will fade, the psychological sequela of being a breast cancer patient, a breast cancer survivor, may also fade with time but will never truly disappear.

Being told that one has breast cancer is unsettling, which is probably the understatement of the ages. Most women with breast cancer report a host of psychological emotions, including fear of death and loss of a sense of control. Feelings of vulnerability and sadness, as well as more psychologically disabling conditions such as clinical depression, anxiety, panic, are not uncommon. Changes in quality of life and interpersonal relationships are also mentioned as being upsetting. It is not just the cancer patient who experiences the trauma of breast cancer treatment. Oftentimes, family and friends are unsure how to react as their loved one/friend undergoes treatment.

The psychological dimensions of adapting to a breast cancer diagnosis naturally vary among individuals. Type and stage of the breast cancer, type of post-op treatment, response to the prescribed treatment (i.e., is the drug regimen "working"?), age at diagnosis, and sociocultural norms will, in some way individually and synergistically, impact coping with the disease. An individual's coping skills, level of emotional maturity, personality characteristics, and social support networks will vary among individuals. Moreover, breast cancer patients' emotional experiences and adjustment in the course of illness vary from one stage to another.[2] For example, the stages of breast cancer can be grouped into three categories: the diagnostic and treatment stage, remission, and recurrence.

The diagnosis and treatment stage demands recognition of the diagnosis of cancer. Denial, anger, fear, anxiety, and depression compete with each other and can affect the most emotionally strong. Coping with the realization that one has cancer, trying to "hold it together" to make important decisions, and enduring the insults of treatment are stressful and, at times, can be overwhelming.

Treatment was successful! You are in remission! It is not uncommon for an individual to experience feelings of increased anxiety when treatment is completed. Am I really "cured"? How shall I resume my life? The periodic checkups are a constant reminder that there may be a risk of recurrence. I could always tell when my mother was going for her follow-up checkups. Her anxiety, which she tried to hide from her daughters, was evident, and the palpable relief when she was told "everything looks good" also was obvious.

Cancer recurrence is the cruelest twist of fate. Coping with this news, this setback, can test the most stalwart. After 15 years in remission, my mother's cancer returned, unleashing a torrent of emotions in her, my sisters, and me. Words cannot express the feelings we collectively and privately felt, but we all agreed that the "best way" forward was to be optimistic and fight the battle (again).

Quality of Life Upended

Undergoing treatment for breast cancer can often feel all consuming. One's life revolves around treatment appointments and medication schedules, leaving little time for "me time." All of this affects quality of life (as defined and perceived by the individual), a subjective phenomenon for which there is no generally agreed definition.[3] Quality of life is often measured as a subjective assessment of health status and well-being that includes physical, psychological, social, and spiritual components.

Since an increasing number of women are surviving for years after their breast cancer diagnosis, issues such as body image, relationships, financial and occupational concerns, and sexual relations are particularly important to address when discussing quality of life and breast cancer during and after treatment. Issues relating to sexuality, reestablishment of intimacy, concerns about dating, and thoughts about becoming pregnant may seem trivial or unimportant during the early phases of treatment, but become more relevant after completion of treatment. Removal of all or part of the breast, hair loss, weight gain, reduction in libido, and sexual dysfunction secondary to estrogen problems stemming from the medication prescribed can impact resumption of sexual relations regardless of the age of the individual.

Understanding the issues related to premature menopause and fertility among younger breast cancer survivors is especially important in light of the fact that more women are delaying childbearing, and a diagnosis of breast cancer complicates things. Chemotherapy, in particular, carries with it reproductive and gynecological implications that younger women may find complicate plans for childbearing. Also, due to the rapid change in menopausal status in chemotherapy-induced ovarian failure, the symptoms of menopause can be more severe than those that occur with natural aging.

Early menopause may also have an adverse impact on sexual functioning. Discussion of fertility and menopause at the time of diagnosis is probably more than a woman can handle. The shock of the diagnosis and the fear of mortality probably overshadow any comprehension of a discussion of fertility-related topics. While it is important to bring up the topic so as to provide information about the short- and long-term gynecological and reproductive sequela of breast cancer treatment, a more in depth discussion about fertility-related issues, premature menopause, and other relevant issues that the patient might have questions about should take place once the individual is undergoing post-op treatment and thinking more clearly about her sexual needs.

Coping Styles

I have heard from cancer survivors that if you have a "will to live" or a "fighting spirit" your chances of survival are increased. Some cancer survivors believe that there is a direct relationship between their psychological state and their long-term survival. Those who seem helpless or hopeless, those who are having difficulty coping with their disease, are thought to have a poorer chance of survival. The literature on this topic is unclear, as some studies found a relationship between mental health symptoms and disease outcome and other did not. So many factors would have to be taken into account before one could draw such a conclusion. While mental health may have some effect on coping with cancer, one would need to know much more about the clinical and preexisting mental health issues of individuals before one could state with any statistical certainly that one's mental health contributes to survival. It may well be the case that those with a more positive attitude cope better than those with a more negative attitude, but to say that mental health contributes in some way to an individual's prognosis is probably stretching things a bit.

For the most part, individual studies looking at psychological factors and cancer survival are not sufficiently rigorous to reach a statistically valid conclusion. Many studies fail to control for important medical and demographic risk factors, which could inflate the importance of those psychological factors that are being studied (and not all studies focus on the same psychological factors, further complicating the issue). Small sample sizes in most of these studies also compromise the ability to detect an affect. In some studies, the participants were self-selected (i.e., they specifically wanted to be part of the study for their own personal reasons) as opposed to a more rigorous randomized study that would eliminate this type of bias. The point I am making is that it is important to understand how the study is designed, who is included in the study, and if there are sufficient number of participants in the study. Flawed study design leads to flawed and misleading findings.

Rather than basing one's conclusion on an individual study, it is preferable to see if a systematic review has been published. Systematic reviews assess the strengths and weaknesses of a large number of studies that have been published on a topic and select only those that meet a rigorous standard for inclusion in the systematic review. In this way, the weaker studies are excluded, ensuring that only the well-designed studies are included. A recent systematic review of studies that focused on psychological coping styles among cancer patients, and how these coping styles influenced or affected survival and/or recurrence, found no statistically significant associations with survival or recurrence by coping styles.[4] Neither a fighting spirit nor feelings of hopelessness/helplessness were shown to have an important part in survival from or recurrence of cancer. The takeaway message is that while coping styles may help an individual deal with her treatment, they are not associated with better survival.

Everyone Is an Individual with Their Own Ways of Coping

Dimensions of psychological distress will vary from person to person; emotional distress such as anxiety, sadness, and depression present in different ways from person to person.

The experience of chemotherapy is a nightmare! Losing control of one's bodily functions, dealing with extreme nausea, and having no energy made me suddenly feel helpless. I felt like I was going to die.

Marsha, age 59, breast cancer survivor

Marsha is probably not alone. Many other breast cancer survivors probably have similar feelings and thoughts and found a way to deal with their situation in a way that made sense to them.

Many breast cancer patients feel overwhelmed by the diagnosis. Marsha goes on to say, "When I was first told that I had breast cancer, many thoughts went through my mind: It can't be true. It can't be happening to me. I feel fine. There must be some mistake." Since a diagnosis of breast cancer, or any cancer for that matter, is a major stressful event, and since life from then on will never be the way it was before the diagnosis, the expression of sadness, distress, or despair could be considered to be a "normal" reaction to the diagnosis.

Many cancer patients feel overwhelmed and are unable to get tasks done as easily as before the diagnosis. Some report that they have little energy and have trouble concentrating. Chemotherapy and radiation can do that to you! Others are unable to concentrate and feel that they are tired all the time. While these symptoms/reactions may be expected as one progresses through treatment, in some cases, they can be an indication of depression. It is important to distinguish depression from sadness or ennui. Depression is much more than feeling sad.

Once the shock of the diagnosis ebbs, new challenges arise, including dealing with the biological and physiological changes associated with treatment. Many cancer medications cause not only physical side effects but also psychological side effects (i.e., mood swings) because of the way they interact with the body's chemistry. Cancer patients stress the importance of having access to information and want to know what to expect at each stage of treatment. How will I feel during and after chemotherapy? How will I feel during and after radiation? What are considered to be "normal" feelings and what are "abnormal" feelings? What should trigger intervention from the medical team? Many cancer patients express the desire for a sense of control over their illness. By and large, when an individual participates, to the desired degree, in a discussion about treatment, a sense of control is enhanced.

Cancer patients also want a sense of reassurance. Support groups provide a crucial source of reassurance. Hearing from others who are going through the same thing is reassuring and helpful. Cancer patients want to feel that family, friends, and the medical team understand her concerns and fears.

What helped me the most is that I was given the names of others who were willing to speak to new patients. My "chemo pal" told me what to expect with the chemotherapy treatments. During radiation treatments, other women spoke about their specific issues. Having access to such support was reassuring and helpful to me. It really helped to talk about what was happening/what was going to happen to me during such a stressful time.

Marsha, age 59, breast cancer survivor

The Importance of Support

The importance of psychological support (informational and emotional) during and after cancer treatment is an important component in the care and recovery process. Support networks, in whatever form, serve as an important source of comfort and offer a sense of reassurance, for example, learning what to expect from treatment or being told that one's emotions/feelings are normal.

The effectiveness of support groups can vary depending on the individual's comfort level in disclosing feelings and concerns as well as the perceived benefit of participating in a group, either in person or online. Many individuals will feel more comfortable sharing their inner thoughts and fears with their spouse, close family, or close friends. That being said, while the medical team is trained to detect changes in mood and can intervene with medication and coping skills to help their patient get over some rough patches, the patient's family, too, will need support and guidance as they cope with the diagnosis and subsequent treatment. The key message is that no patient or her family should feel that they individually and collectively have to deal with her cancer alone. The following chapter presents much more information on support groups.

Fear of Recurrence

What stays in my mind is always the question: Will my cancer come back? When? I am a high risk cancer survivor, so I am well aware that this [fear of recurrence] will always be with me.

Marsha, age 59, breast cancer survivor

At some point, the chemo and/or radiation treatments will end. This will mark a time of psychological adjustment. Yet, there will be constant reminders of the disease (physical and perhaps mental) in the form of anniversary dates and follow-up checkups. Probably the biggest threat to psychological well-being is cancer recurrence. More than a decade after the date of her initial diagnosis, my mother received the devastating news that her cancer had recurred. I cannot explain the psychological jolt we all felt when we heard that news. And Marsha, who has been quoted in this chapter, was told 10 years after her initial diagnosis that her breast cancer *might* have recurred. Fortunately for her it was a false alarm, but she now lives with an uneasy feeling that her cancer could indeed return.

Breast cancer has the potential to spread to almost any region of the body, although the most common sites include the bone, lung, brain, or liver. There are three types of recurrent breast cancer: local (cancerous tumor cells remain in the original site only to reappear at a later time), regional (the cancer has spread from the original site), and distant (the cancer has metastasized to other parts of the body). A recurrence of noninvasive breast cancer is far less serious than a recurrence of invasive cancer. Distant recurrence is a serious matter, and the survival rate is considerably lower than that for women whose cancer is confined to the breast or axillary nodes. Besides local and regional recurrences, a new cancer may occur years after the initial cancer diagnosis.

More often than not, the diagnosis of recurrent cancer is more devastating or psychologically difficult for a woman than her initial breast cancer diagnosis. Those with recurrence have fears and concerns different from those experienced at first diagnosis. Feelings of injustice, discouragement, hopelessness, and despair are commonly cited. The emotional roller coaster of coping with the recurrence, as well as the recognition of one's mortality, is hugely stressful for the patient and her family. My mother felt betrayed when, 15 years after her initial battle with breast cancer, she was diagnosed with advanced, metastatic, distant recurrence. The anger of having to undergo chemotherapy and radiation again made her furious. But she never gave up her fight until three months before her death, when the rapidly spreading cancer finally sapped her will to live.

What Is Psycho-Oncology?

The medical team's response to the patient's emotional needs is as important as addressing the physical/clinical aspects of care. A clearly explained, individually tailored delivery of information by the physician can do much to help allay patient fears and anxiety. Implicit in this, however, is that the physician is able to discern and detect a patient's need for emotional support. Unfortunately, many physicians do not properly elicit their patients' emotional concerns. They are far more comfortable dealing with the clinical aspects of care as well as meeting the direct informational needs of their patients rather than dealing with the psychological issues that certainly accompany cancer care.

Of course, the extent and severity of psychological symptoms will vary greatly among patients, but it is rare that a patient would not suffer from some psychological fallout from her disease. Complicating the issue is that not every patient feels comfortable disclosing or discussing her emotional problems directly to her physician. Some perceive doctors as busy people who should not be bothered with their worries or fears. Others may feel that their worries are "normal" under the circumstances; therefore, the doctor should not be "bothered." Those with a more fatalistic attitude may feel that an emotional response to their cancer is reflective of their belief that nothing can be done about it anyway and, as such, are reluctant to share their feelings. Among those who do not want to be seen as uncooperative or ungrateful, these individuals might be more likely to allude indirectly to their emotional needs rather than to directly express their feelings.

Given that there are different ways of expressing emotion, it is important that the medical team be astute in picking up on nonverbal cues such as body language and body posture and to reach out to those who are unable to express their emotional concerns directly. The reality is that patient and physician behavior influence how well a patient's emotional needs, no matter how trivial, are detected and addressed. Being attentive to facial expressions, posture, and other indirect cues can help the medical team raise the issue of emotional need. It may be that the patient is more comfortable raising the issue with the nurse, not the doctor, which is fine so long as the medical team follows up. The nurse is a pivotal person on the team and is usually the one to find out how distressed the patient is and what kind of problems she is dealing with.

Since an overwhelming majority of women are surviving for years if not decades after being diagnosed with breast cancer, addressing the psychological issues of survivorship is an important part of the process of regaining physical and mental health. Recognizing the importance of and need for psychological support during and after cancer treatment, the medical profession understood the value of developing a specialty area that would deal with the myriad of psychiatric and psychological issues stemming from cancer therapy. The need for mental health support is particularly important to help the patient and her family cope with the stress and anxiety of being a cancer patient.

The subspecialty of psycho-oncology began formally in the mid-1970s, around the same time that the stigma of talking about cancer faded, making it more acceptable to talk with a patient about her disease and the implications thereof. Psycho-oncology focuses on the social, behavioral, and ethical aspects of cancer. It addresses the psychological responses of patients to cancer at all stages of the disease, as well as that of their families and the providers to care.[5] It is a multidisciplinary field that includes, surgery, medicine, oncology, nursing, pediatrics, radiotherapy, epidemiology, immunology, endocrinology, pathology, bioethics, and psychiatry. Working collaboratively, the objective is to have the medical team assess and treat psychological reactions at all stages of the cancer as well as the stresses on the family and also the clinical staff. Figure 11.1 illustrates the many dimensions of psycho-oncology.

Members of the caregiving team provide education, counseling, and referrals when warranted to patients and their family to discuss issues of concern, develop coping strategies, help the patient regain a sense of control over her life, and work toward improving quality of life. There is no one treatment plan that should be adopted. Rather, an individual assessment of needs and wants should be done so as to design the most appropriate plan of action *at the time*, with the understanding that things will and do change, which will necessitate reviewing and refining a plan that would meet needs and wants *at that time*.

Reach Out to Other Professionals for Advice

In addition to addressing the psychological needs of the patient, financial counseling also might be an important component of the healing process. The costs of cancer treatment is substantial, and an individual's personal financial burden to pay for care could be quite high regardless of whether she has health insurance or not.[6] It is not the primary role of the clinician to focus on the financial aspects of care. A financial counselor is well equipped to answer questions about financial issues relating to medical treatment. Further, as the breast cancer survivor works on her medical issues, it might be a good time to take a fresh look at one's will and estate planning. Lawyers, especially trust and estate lawyers, will help with legal issues to ensure that proper inheritance issues are in place.

End Note

The diagnosis and treatment of breast cancer is a stressful time for both the patient and her family. Changes in behavior and mood are common. Many women experience a host of psychological symptoms at some point during the course of treatment and posttreatment, including but not limited to sleep disturbance, fatigue, stress, anxiety, irritability, inability to cope, sadness, and depression. Feelings of loss of control can be upending and upsetting.

The good news is that today breast cancer has shifted from being perceived as a fatal illness to one that is similar to a chronic disease. As with hypertension or diabetes, typical chronic diseases, the majority of those diagnosed with breast cancer will live for years after their initial diagnosis. And this makes it even more imperative that the individual receive the "best" possible treatment for the disease as well as for her mental health. The provision of optimal care requires the use of a multidisciplinary team that,

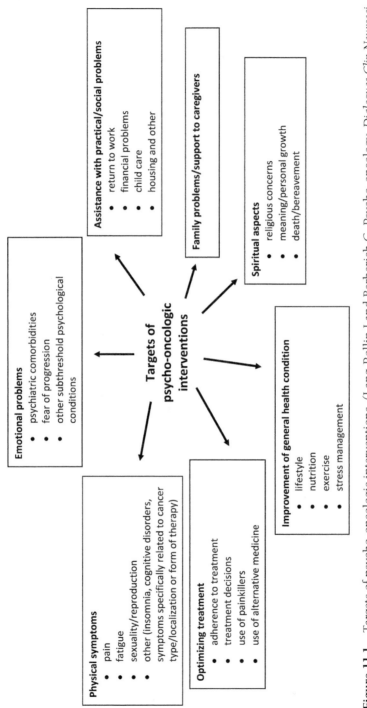

Physical symptoms
- pain
- fatigue
- sexuality/reproduction
- other (insomnia, cognitive disorders, symptoms specifically related to cancer type/localization or form of therapy)

Optimizing treatment
- adherence to treatment
- treatment decisions
- use of painkillers
- use of alternative medicine

Emotional problems
- psychiatric comorbidities
- fear of progression
- other subthreshold psychological conditions

Targets of psycho-oncologic interventions

Improvement of general health condition
- lifestyle
- nutrition
- exercise
- stress management

Assistance with practical/social problems
- return to work
- financial problems
- child care
- housing and other

Family problems/support to caregivers

Spiritual aspects
- religious concerns
- meaning/personal growth
- death/bereavement

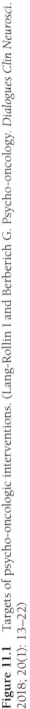

Figure 11.1 Targets of psycho-oncologic interventions. (Lang-Rollin I and Berberich G. Psycho-oncology. *Dialogues Clin Neurosci.* 2018; 20(1): 13–22)

importantly, includes mental health professionals and makes use of support networks.

No cancer patient should have to manage her psychological feelings alone in a vacuum. The medical team should be able to work with the patient to address these issues. For many, the ability to regain a sense of control over one's life may take time, but with the help of the medical team, family, and friends, a sense of control and confidence can be achieved.

CHAPTER TWELVE

Physicians and Patients Need to Communicate with Each Other

Medicine is an art whose magic and creative ability have long been recognized as residing in the interpersonal aspects of patient-physician relationship.[1]

The tremendous advances in diagnosis and treatment of breast cancer that have occurred over the past few decades have truly revolutionized how cancer care is delivered. The science that has led to these advances continues, providing clinicians with many more options in their treatment arsenal to consider than was possible even a few years ago. Yet, an important (and sometimes overlooked) component of treatment decision-making is the patient. Physicians need to be cognizant of the importance of including the patient in decision-making and to embrace and encourage the individual to be an engaged and active participant in her own care. Decision-making should not be a one-way street. Shared decision-making, a critical feature in a good doctor-patient relationship, refers to the physician and patient arriving at a specific course of action based on a common understanding of the goals of treatment and the risks and benefits of the chosen treatment.

The issue of shared decision-making and the doctor-patient relationship has been discussed in the literature repeatedly for many years. Yet, only fairly recently has the medical profession started to take action to understand and acknowledge that asking patients how much they want to be involved in decisions regarding treatment is an important foundation for an informed, collaborative relationship. Patients do want to be involved in, or at the very least, informed about, health care decisions that will impact their course of treatment. Doing so does make a difference, as this chapter will explore.

Doctor Knows Best Paternalism

Historically, throughout medical school and residency training, medical students and young doctors in training were advised to maintain a clinical distance and not to get too emotionally involved with patients, to keep an emotional distance so as to protect themselves. This was especially so with treating cancer patients. Physicians saw themselves as father figures (the overwhelming majority of physicians in the 19th and 20th centuries were males) whose role was to make decisions about medical care that they thought was best for the patient. The "paternalistic" physician presented information in a selective manner that encouraged the patient to assent to the doctor's decision. Patients were expected to adhere to the doctor's plan and not to ask too many questions, and for the most part, the patient was in no position not to go along with the doctor's recommendations since the patient did not have the knowledge or training to even think of questioning the doctor. That was just not done.

In 1984, Jay Katz wrote *The Silent World of the Doctor and Patient*, in which he argued compassionately for the ability of patients to participate in treatment decisions.[2] In the book, Dr. Katz relates the story of Iphigenia Jones, a breast cancer patient he met while attending a panel discussion. Ms. Jones was a 21-year-old attractive, single woman who developed a malignant breast lesion. Her surgeon (a male) strongly believed that breast-conserving surgery with radiation was an inferior treatment and scheduled her for a mastectomy without discussing any alternative with Ms. Jones, as was the common practice at the time. In the days leading up to the surgery, however, Ms. Jones's surgeon became increasingly anxious about performing a grossly scarring procedure on such a young woman. The night before the surgery, the surgeon (finally—author emphasis) had a conversation with Ms. Jones in which he defended his belief that a mastectomy was the best option; yet, he also discussed breast-conserving options. Ms. Jones decided against having a mastectomy, and after taking time to educate herself about viable options, she opted for lumpectomy with radiation. Had her surgeon not have a crisis of conscience, Ms. Jones most certainly would have undergone a mastectomy. She would have had no idea that there were other options that should have been presented and considered. The preceding story illustrates in a personal way the importance of keeping open lines of communication between the doctor and the patient and involving the patient in the decision-making process.

Dr. Barron Lerner, a physician-ethicist, in his eloquent book *The Good Doctor* beautifully discusses his perspective of the art of medicine, the importance of doctors knowing their patients beyond the physical ailments, and tailoring treatments to individual patients to do what was best for them. He writes that the era of doctors keeping patients and their families in the dark, making life-and-death decisions without them (or their next of kin), is what the bioethics movement sought to change.[3]

Patient-Centered Care and Shared Decision-Making

There are several different theories and models for medical decision-making that have been proposed: the doctor-centered approach and the patient-centered approach being the two prominent ones. The former, essentially a thing of the past, affirms that the doctor is an expert whose task it is to make the decisions for the patient. In contrast, the patient-centered approach includes the patient, who plays an active role in the decision-making process. The doctor, with his or her knowledge and expertise, talks with (as opposed to talking to or talking at) the patient and helps guide the decision-making discussion. The focus is to empower the patient to be an active and engaged partner in the dialogue. The patient is encouraged to ask questions, and the doctor needs to provide answers in a way that the patient can understand. Moreover, the doctor needs to incorporate the values and expectations of the patient when making treatment recommendations, taking into account not only the patient's wishes but also the patient's family and social and religious factors. More on this later. The following diagram illustrates the interrelationship between doctor and patient in shared decision-making.

This new egalitarian approach of shared decision-making affirms that the patient should play as active a role as comfortable in the decision-making process, which is especially important in the care of breast cancer patients. A 35-year-old mother with young children is very likely to have different concerns and expectations about her breast cancer treatment than an older woman who has already raised her family. Each has concerns and fears, but their perspective will probably be different because of their different stage of life.

Fostering a patient-centered, shared decision-making approach to care for cancer patients is more complicated than that for patients with other potentially less serious illnesses.[4] Providing care to the cancer patient involves multiple treatment modalities, including chemotherapy, radiation, and surgery, all of which need to be coordinated among different cancer care specialists. For example, women with breast cancer can often choose from different courses of treatment (i.e., mastectomy vs lumpectomy, radiation and/or chemo, different medication options). Treatment regimens are usually time intensive, debilitating, and often result in serious and sometimes long-term complications. Patient understanding and comprehension of instructions given by the medical team is especially important.

In the primary care setting, many studies have shown that there can be confusion and misunderstanding about what the physician and the medical team say during the medical encounter, leading to miscommunication between doctor and patient. Depending on the complexity of the information imparted, patients with more serious conditions tend not to register what is being said to them. This is certainly true among cancer patients. Studies have shown repeatedly that once an individual is told that she has cancer, there is little to no information that is retained after receiving the diagnosis. For this reason, individuals are encouraged to bring a family member or trusted friend to the appointment to act as a scribe, recording information that can then be discussed with the patient once the reality of the situation has sunk in. A physician who goes into a lengthy discourse of treatment options and prognosis with a newly diagnosed cancer patient is essentially wasting his or her time. The patient is not going to retain much from the conversation. All the patient hears and remembers is that she has cancer.

Patients, regardless of their medical issue, undoubtedly do not have the sufficient clinical knowledge that the physician has. While this is understood by both doctor and patient, another factor has to be taken into account so as to ensure that the information and instructions imparted by the health care team is understood by the patient: the issue of health literacy. An individual's level of health literacy (as defined by the Institute of Medicine as the degree to which individuals have the capacity to obtain, process, and understand basic health information and services needed to make appropriate health decisions) can complicate shared decision-making. It is estimated that over one-third of the U.S. adult population (approximately 80 million individuals) have poor health literacy, which is most notably prevalent in older adults, racial and ethnic minority populations, individuals for whom English is a second language, those who have not completed high school, and people living in poverty.[5] With cancer, even those with good health literacy may not retain important information if they feel overwhelmed with new terminology while grappling with a diagnosis of cancer and all of the information the doctor is trying to explain.[6]

There are numerous organizations that have prepared easily understood, accurate information on cancer, cancer prognosis, treatment benefits and harms, palliative care, and psychosocial support. These resources should be made available to the patient and her family and by so doing more likely than not improve patient-centered communication and shared decision-making. Further, decisions often need to be reassessed throughout the treatment process, depending on how the patient is responding to the cancer care. The emotional, financial, and logistical repercussions of a cancer diagnosis and the complexity of treatment options, together with patients' limitations in health literacy, can make it difficult for patients and their families to actively engage in making health care decisions. Figure 12.1 illustrates the components of patient-centered care.

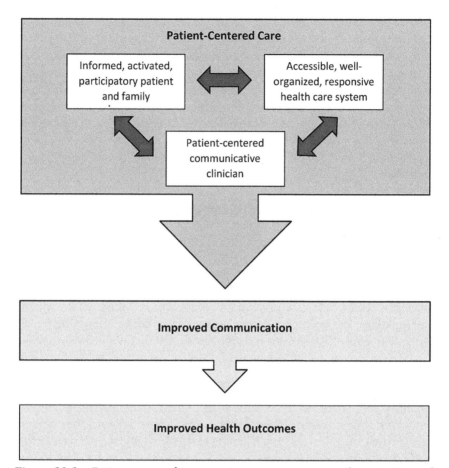

Figure 12.1 Patient-centered communication in cancer care (Epstein RM and Street RL, Jr. Patient-centered communication in cancer care: Promoting healing and reducing suffering. National Cancer Institute, 2007. NIH Publication No. 07-6225)

There is ample evidence to show that decision-making can be improved through use of decision aids, tools that provide patients with evidence-based, objective information on all treatment options for a given condition. Decision aids can include written material, web-based tools, videos, and multimedia programs. Each is designed to facilitate patient understanding of treatment options and enable patients to take a more active role in decision-making. Some aids can be used by the patient only and others by physician and/or care team with the patient. Selecting the "best" aid might be a daunting task, as it is estimated that there are more than 500 decision aids currently available![7] Adjuvant!Online, for example, is one of the more popular of the decision aids available.

In summary, each patient should be treated individually, as patients often have very different expectations regarding the amount of information they need in order to make shared decisions about their care. Some individuals will want to know as much as possible, while others may not. This can present a challenge to the physician as well as the care team. Physicians need to appreciate the range of patient and family needs in order to create a healthy doctor-patient relationship and must take care not to misjudge patient preferences.

Shared Decision-Making Requires Good Listening Skills

The shift from paternalism in the medical encounter to a system that encourages active patient participation in shared decision-making has been hailed as an important improvement in building trust in the doctor-patient relationship as well as in the way the two parties communicate with each other. Physicians today are under a lot of stress to be "efficient" during the medical exam, and doctors often rely on automatic, fast thinking when interacting with patients. However, research has shown that physicians who take the time to actively listen to patients have stronger relationships with their patients.

Listening also conveys a sense of respect. From the physician perspective, an important part of medicine is listening to the patient describe her symptoms, concerns, and fears. Unfortunately, it is frequently heard that patients perceive that their doctor is not listening to them, is ignoring their concerns, or is not taking what they say seriously. For some, there can be a distressing lack of communication with the doctor, which negatively affects not only the relationship but also, in some cases, the clinical course of treatment (i.e., poor patient compliance, misunderstandings). Listening to the patient without judgment, interruption, or preconceptions can be difficult for many physicians who have a myriad of other things on their mind, but it is an essential tool in the practice of medicine.

A doctor who listens to his or her patient will undoubtedly pick up on patient fears, anxiety, needs, and wants and, with his or her knowledge and expertise, will be in a much better position to help guide the patient in shared decision-making. The doctor's challenge is to figure out how to empower the patient to be an active and engaged partner in the dialogue. The patient should be encouraged to ask questions, and the doctor needs to provide answers in a way that the patient can understand. Moreover, the doctor needs to incorporate the values and expectations of the patient when making treatment recommendations, taking into account not only the patient's wishes but also those of the patient's family (hopefully they will be similar if not the same as that of the patient). Sociocultural beliefs and religious factors also must be taken into consideration in the shared decision-making process.

Attentive listening skills, empathy, and use of open-ended questions are some examples of skillful communication. Dr. Danielle Ofri's book *What Patients Say, What Doctors Hear*[8] provides insight into factors that contribute to physician-patient communication breakdowns and medical errors and discusses the challenges that doctors and patients face in communicating and provides optimistic insights on how to improve health care. In her book, she stresses that listening and communication skills are powerful tools for patient care.

In this digital age, harnessing the power of technology can do much to help patients remember what was said to them by their doctor. A simple cell phone recording enables a patient to better remember important information or to share it with family member. Authors of a recent study on digital recordings reported that 1 in 10 patients record doctors' visits, usually on a cell phone.[9] While the potential benefits of digital recordings are enormous, there are also serious implications for consent procedures, privacy, and cyber security, the authors say. For example, harvesting data from patient recordings of doctors' visits could become a viable commercial prospect. Facebook has already declared an interest in health-related data. DeepMind, a Google-owned artificial intelligence company, acquired vast amounts of data from patients without their consent. Balancing the potential benefits of digital recordings with the potential harms to privacy is something that must be worked out before things get out of hand.

How to Break Bad News to Patients in the Digital Age

How a doctor frames "bad news" can have lasting implications for the doctor-patient relationship. Delivering bad news is one of the most daunting tasks faced by physicians. Medical schools do not, in general, do a very good job of teaching how to give bad news. Many studies have looked at this issue, all with similar results. One study, for example, found that that 93% of physician respondents perceived delivering bad news to be a very important skill with 7% stating that it was a somewhat important skill; however, only 43% of respondents felt they had the training to effectively deliver such news.[10] While the consensus is that a physician should be empathetic, make an effort to truly understand the patient's perspective, keep things simple and easy to understand, and be available should the patient have follow-up questions, in reality, physicians acknowledge that they fall short in achieving this objective. Around 85% of physicians polled on the subject of breaking bad news said that they needed additional training to be effective when delivering bad news.[11]

Another important component in the breaking bad news toolbox is to have the patient verify to the best of her ability the material presented by the doctor. Verification techniques are an invaluable, often overlooked tool for improving patient comprehension of bad news. Physicians can verify that their patients have an understanding of the information that is being told to them by asking the patient to restate in their own words what it is that the doctor has told them. Verification can help avoid many of the miscommunications that can result when a patient tries to translate "doctor speak" to everyday language. And this is also true for correcting any misinformation the patient may have after doing an Internet search of their illness.

Communication and Patient Satisfaction

Good doctor-patient communication also impacts patient satisfaction, an important quality indicator used by just about every medical center to gauge how well it is doing. An open and trusting relationship has been shown to be correlated with patient satisfaction, another important component in the doctor-patient relationship.

Today, patients want doctors who can skillfully diagnose and treat their sicknesses as well as communicate with them effectively. Doctors are expected to be forthcoming with their patients concerning their medical condition and treatment options. As patients are drawn into the decision-making process, and acknowledging the imbalance in knowledge between doctor and patient, it is imperative for the doctor to explain the patient's medical condition in laymen terms and present options (pros and cons of each) so that the doctor and the patient, as a team, can agree on a plan of action. When a doctor and patient agree about the nature of the treatment, studies have shown a strong association with recovery.[12] Numerous studies also have been published showing that a more patient-centric encounter results in improved patient and doctor satisfaction. Everyone wins![13]

It may seem intuitive to anyone who has been to the doctor that satisfaction (however defined by the patient) can influence the quality of the visit. Physicians who take time to listen, to answer questions, to show that "they care" are often viewed as being a "good doctor." Patients pick up on how the doctor is talking to them (i.e., tone of voice, words that are used) as well as nonverbal cues such as posture and body language. Is the doctor nervous? Irritated? Aggressive in manner? Or is the doctor friendly? Attentive? A verbal/nonverbal mismatch on the part of the physician can be perceived as a lack of genuineness and can lead to patient dissatisfaction and distrust.

Ability to communicate in the same language can also serve to create a communication barrier, which impacts the doctor-patient relationship, shared decision-making, and patient satisfaction. Explaining treatment options, obtaining patient consent for treatment, and explaining the potential risks and benefits of treatment are hard enough, but trying to communicate these in the language that is spoken by the patient makes things even harder. Clearly, the way a physician communicates risk can affect a patient's perception of risk. The cultural background of the doctor, the medical team, and the patient will influence communication. Cultural sensitivity is an essential prerequisite for building an effective doctor-patient relationship. Taking into account cultural norms and beliefs is very important when discussing options with a patient for whom English is her second language. Those patients who do not speak or understand English present greater challenges, and there must be someone on the team who can serve as translator during office visits.

The main independent predictors of satisfaction have been patients' perceptions of communication and partnership with her doctor. Good communication tends to be linked with the patient's satisfaction with the care she is getting as well as how well the patient is adhering to treatment regimens. Poor communication can lead to unnecessary misunderstandings that promote distrust, anger, and possibly legal action. I often tell my medical students that patients are much less likely to sue if they like their doctor regardless of how competent the doctor actually is! A superior doctor with lousy bedside manners is more likely to be sued by a disgruntled patient compared to a less superior doctor who has a wonderful bedside manner. It pays to be nice, kind, and be a good listener—it also helps if the doctor is also good at his or her craft, but that may not be "good enough" if the patient perceives that the doctor doesn't really communicate well.

How to Get the Patient to Comply with Treatment

Constructive, open lines of communication between doctors and patients have an impact on patient compliance with instructions. Many studies have looked at physician communication skills and their relationship to patient compliance and patient outcomes. In general, the likelihood that a patient will comply with instructions is a function of the patient's perceived benefits of the intervention weighted against the costs and potential side effects of the treatment. Patient noncompliance with cancer treatment, similar to compliance with treatment for long-term chronic disease, has consequences. Not complying with treatment can lead to complications and even death.

There are some cancer patients who seek nontraditional types of therapies, including complementary and alternative medicine (CAM), in hopes of gaining time or even a cure. Having a dialogue with the doctor is important because some of these therapies are known to be not effective or, worse, could be dangerous. Some physicians may view CAM as a form of noncompliance, while the patient may feel that CAM offers some degree of hope. Steve Jobs, founder of Apple, was diagnosed with a rare form of pancreatic cancer in 2003. He allegedly delayed surgery to remove the tumor, the recommended treatment, during which he attempted to treat his cancer with alternative medicine, including a special diet and CAM therapies, including acupuncture and botanicals. After a delay of nine months after diagnosis, Mr. Jobs opted for surgery, but he died seven years later.[14]

An open line of communication is necessary for both parties to share their thoughts and collectively arrive at a decision. But not telling the doctor about the types of CAM therapies could lead to potentially serious adverse events and could jeopardize the ability of medical treatment to work effectively. Some botanicals and biologics negatively interact with the prescribed treatment, and the doctor must be aware of the types of CAM the patient is relying on.

Can Doctors Be Taught to Be Good Listeners?

Medical school does an excellent job in teaching soon-to-be doctors about anatomy, clinical diagnosis, and clinical treatments, but can individuals be taught how to listen to and how to communicate with their patients? As noted several times in this chapter, physicians need to listen to patient concerns, and interrupting the patient (which is done frequently by doctors, perhaps unconsciously) does not constitute listening carefully. There have been numerous studies to show convincingly that doctor-patient listening and communicating (but not dominating the conversation) leads to focused, efficient, and patient-centered care.[15]

Of course, it is in the best interest of both doctors and patients that each party understands the importance of listening and communicating with each other. For doctors, this understanding will help them meet the therapeutic and emotional needs of their patients. For patients, this understanding will encourage them to share important information and to ask questions and share concerns with their caregiver. In shared decision-making, the patient leads in areas where she is an expert (i.e., symptoms, preferences, concerns), and the doctor leads in areas where he or she is an expert (i.e., explanation of the disease, treatment options, prognosis). A strong doctor-patient relationship is an important, if not necessary, ingredient in decision-making and often leads to greater patient satisfaction with her care and trust in her doctor's judgment.

Listening to one's patient takes time, and in this age of managed health care, time is a precious commodity. How physicians use clinic time has important implications for quality of care and patient trust.[16] One study (among many on the topic) found that the average length of a doctor visit was 17.4 minutes, with a median of 15.7 minutes. The median talk time by patient was 5.3 minutes and by physician 5.2 minutes. The median time during which neither part spoke was 55 seconds. The average number of topics in a visit was 6.5 (i.e., clinical and psychosocial issues, personal habits, patient initiated topics, and small talk). On average, patients got about 11 seconds to explain the reasons for their visit before they were interrupted by their doctor. Also, studies have found that on average only one in three doctors provides their patients with adequate opportunity to describe their situation.[17] Findings from these studies do not take into account the time the patient spent with the nurse discussing prescribed treatment and answering remaining questions. Use of nonphysician staff saves time for the physician who can then move on to the next patient while helping the patient understand better the nature of her disease and what to expect from the treatment.

Are Women Doctors Better Communicators than Male Doctors?

Does the gender of the doctor make a difference in doctor-patient communication relationships? I have heard it said by many patients that female doctors are better listeners than male doctors and that female doctors tend to care more than their male counterparts. Differences in the interpersonal style of women compared to men are well documented, but that certainly does not mean that only female doctors are sympathetic, kind caregivers. There most probably are plenty of insensitive female physicians, just as there are many male doctors who have wonderful interpersonal skills and are excellent communicators. That being said, there are studies to show that in general female physicians engage in significantly more active partnership behaviors, positive talk, psychological counseling, and emotionally focused talk than their male counterparts. While I am certainly not advocating that female physicians make better doctors than male physicians, or that one should only seek care from a female physician, the point is that there are differences in doctor-patient communication depending on the gender of the patient and the physician.

Are Primary Care Doctors "Better" Listeners than Specialists?

Does the physician's specialty make a difference in time spent listening to the patient? Patients who are referred to a specialist, or who seek care on their own from a specialist, are seeking care for a specific problem (i.e., going to a surgeon or to an endocrinologist for diabetes care). While the specialist also has to take a history and do a physical, including running tests, the need to listen to the patient is as important for the specialist as it is for the primary care physician. While the focus is on the specific medical issue that brought the patient to the specialist in the first place, the specialist still needs to develop a relationship with the patient, and this includes listening to and communicating with the patient: What are the patient's specific concerns related to the condition and to its management? What results are the patient hoping for?

Are specialists "better" listeners than primary care doctors? The short answer is that it probably depends on the individual regardless of the subspecialty.

While it may seem as if the doctor visit has gotten shorter, studies show that this is not necessarily the case. Doctors' visits have actually not gotten appreciably shorter on average over the past decades. In 1992, approximately 70% of doctor visits lasted 15 minutes or less; by 2010, about half were that short.[18] One might ask how the 15-minute visit took hold. Essentially, a 1992 complex formula, the "relative value unit," or RVU, was adopted by Medicare as a standard way to calculate doctors' fees. Based on this formula, a typical primary care office visit should be 1.3 RVUs, which using the American Medical Association coding guidelines at the time translated to 15 minutes. Medicare's reimbursement rules were then adopted by the private insurance companies, and the 15-minute visit became the norm for reimbursing doctors. Of course, more complex visits were allotted more than 15 minutes, and doctors were reimbursed at a higher rate for these visits.

Do short visits (i.e., less than 15 minutes) leave the patient feeling less satisfied with the care rendered? The answer to this question will depend on many factors, including the patient's expectations, the relationship she has with her doctor, the nature of her condition/disease, and probably other intangible factors. What one wants to avoid, regardless of the amount of time of the office visit, is having the patient leave the office frustrated or not satisfied with the physician encounter.

Cancer Patients Have Special Needs

Despite the increasing importance of open communication in cancer care, the literature shows that cancer patients, in particular, have unique needs and concerns in speaking with their oncologists, especially in understanding what the doctor is saying and feeling comfortable in asking questions. Women newly diagnosed with breast cancer have many questions. Am I going to die? How far has the cancer spread? What are my odds for a cure? What are my treatment options? How am I going to feel once I start treatment? Given the huge variability among breast cancer patients (i.e., different age, ethnicity, educational level, socioeconomic background, etc.), issues and concerns will naturally need to be tailored to the individual. Younger women, for example, might be more concerned about issues related to sexuality and physical attractiveness during and after treatment. Older women might be more concerned about issues of self-care. Feelings of resignation might be more prevalent in some women, while others may approach cancer treatment as a battle to win at all costs.

For the most part, cancer patients have a strong desire for information about their disease. Patients who engage in active question asking are more likely to build a strong relationship with their doctor and medical team. People who ask more questions get more answers, and these answers help the individual understand better their disease, treatment options, and prognosis. Similarly, individuals who do some research on the nature of their disease can be more informed participants and play a more active role in decision-making. The following quote from one patient sums up this point nicely.

> *My experience has been that if you want to have better communication with your doctor, you have to be informed. You can't go in expecting the doctors or the nurses to solve all the problems and have all the answers for you. I think you make it easier for the [medical team] if you take it on yourself to learn something about your [treatment].*[19]

Yet, the desire for more information can be sometimes confused with a presumed wish to participate in clinical decision-making. How active a partner in decision-making the woman elects to be is another story. The important message is that doctors should not assume that whether a patient asks a lot of questions, or doesn't, she isn't interested in having a role in decision-making.

Another factor, health status, can influence decision-making preferences for women with breast cancer. Women with benign breast disease and women with malignant breast disease have different concerns and needs. Studies have shown that healthy (i.e., benign breast disease) women are more likely to be more active in the decision-making process, whereas women with malignant breast disease, especially those in the end stages of breast cancer, are more passive partners in decision-making. As was stated many times in previous chapters, one size does not fit all.

There are other factors that can contribute to strained doctor-patient communication in treating cancer patients. Physicians who care for cancer patients may themselves experience tremendous psychological distress. Oncologists are managing relationships with patients who are doing their best to cope with a serious and potentially fatal disease. As a result, oncologists may consciously or unconsciously create a professional detachment from their cancer patient. Distancing tactics could damage the relationship with the patient and her family. Further, by trying to ease anxiety and distress, oncologists could decide to withhold information that they feel may not be necessary to share at that time. Doctors' personal feelings of unease or anxiety over the uncertainties of cancer care also may influence the amount of information given to the patient and her family.

Doctors, in general, are not comfortable discussing end-of-life care with their terminally ill patient. The doctor's feelings of powerlessness or failure to be able to do much for the patient may create an awkward, distant relationship. The key is for all involved to talk to each other openly and honestly about what would be the "best" course of action in the short term so that planning for the long term can be accomplished based on a solid foundation of shared decision-making.

It takes a team of medical and health professionals to care for a breast cancer patient: an internist, oncologist, radiation oncologist, breast surgeon, anesthesiologist, oncology nurses, social worker, physician assistant, medical technicians, clinical nurse specialist, nurse case manager, dietitian/nutritionist, dosimetrist (the individual who calculates and plans the correct dose of radiation therapy), pain specialist, occupational therapist, physical therapist, palliative care team, mental health specialists, and probably others that I did not think of. Navigating this daunting array of health care professionals can be both confusing and potentially stressful for the patient. The possibility of miscommunication and lack of continuity among the care giving team is something that needs to be considered. Some patients get the sense that they have lost control over their own care and that nobody is in charge.

> *I began to feel like a number or nameless person. I felt like there wasn't any recognition of individuality. There was a medical protocol that was being followed, but I felt like I didn't have any input or control. At times I felt a bit patronized or condescended to.*[20]

Successfully navigating the medical team requires that patients understand the different roles of the team. There needs to be someone in charge who can deal with the patient's questions, concerns, fears. Usually a nurse case manager fulfills that role, and he or she works closely with the others on the medical team to ensure that everyone is on the same page.

The difficulty in maintaining the continuity of the doctor-patient relationship in the context of the multidisciplinary medical team has led to thinking about better ways to provide care to cancer patients. The "one-stop" breast cancer clinics, for example, are a means to bring the team together so as to make it easier for the patient to receive the necessary care from the team in one place and for the individual members of the medical team to communicate with each other in one place. Not only does the "one-stop" care center help streamline patient care, but it also serves to help ease patient anxiety by obviating the need to make multiple visits, usually at different locations, to receive care.

Cancer centers have invested heavily in collaborative interdisciplinary breast cancer specialty centers. For example, the Evelyn H. Lauder Breast Center at the Memorial Sloan Kettering Cancer Center in New York City provides comprehensive breast cancer services that go beyond the standard of care, offering prevention, diagnosis, treatment, and support (i.e., integrative medicine, rehabilitation, survivorship, psychiatry, social work, nutrition, and sexual health), in one dedicated center. Similar "one-stop shopping" cancer centers are provided by other hospitals across the country. These centers, also known as patient-centered oncology medical homes, enable the medical and social service team to easily communicate with each other and provide comprehensive, integrated cancer care under "one roof".

Concluding Thoughts

The patient will never care how much you know, until they know how much you care.[21]

There are things that physicians can do to ensure a good doctor-patient relationship, one built on trust and open communication. Maintaining an open dialogue between doctor and patient is particularly important in cancer care where the emotional strain on the patient, and often on the physician, can be high. A good doctor-patient open line of communication can help allay fears, enhance understanding of the disease and the treatment, and ensure compliance with treatment. Patient satisfaction is also a component of a good doctor-patient relationship, as patients who are more satisfied with their doctor and the care team tend to be more compliant with treatment and more likely to ask questions to help them deal with their illness.

Breast cancer patients have a diverse range of preferences regarding how active a role they wish to play when discussing and choosing treatment options. Whereas many may wish to have a collaborative role in decision-making, others may be more comfortable in a more passive role, letting the physician and care team take the lead in managing decisions related to treatment options. Some patients are assertive, ask a lot of questions, come prepared with information obtained from the Internet, and want to be seen as an active and engaged partner in the relationship. Others are not comfortable in such a role. Perhaps an ideal model would be a combination of both, where the patient would take a more active stance in areas where she is an expert (i.e., her symptoms, concerns), and the physician leads in areas where he or she is an expert (i.e., treatment options). Regardless, physicians should encourage their patients to ask questions and make appropriate referrals in cases where the patient is having difficulty coping with her illness. The patient should understand that there is a team dedicated to helping her at every stage of her illness.

The physician, the care team, and the patient need to communicate in a way that facilitates a good doctor-patient relationship. Physicians should not "talk down" to their patients; should not use medical terms without explaining their meaning in a way that the patient can understand; and should not ignore or dismiss patients' concerns, fears, and anxieties. In turn, patients should be open and honest in conveying their feelings so that the physician and care team can make sure to address these issues during the medical visit. Neither the physician and the care team nor the patient are mind readers. They need to talk to each other and work as a team. Mutual understanding is important to help the patient get through what is often a grueling course of treatment as well as post-treatment ongoing care.

CHAPTER THIRTEEN

You Are Not Alone: Support Groups and Online Forums for Cancer Patients

Dealing with a diagnosis of breast cancer, its subsequent treatment, and the psychological sequela should not be done in a vacuum. Support from family, friends, and the medical team is so important during all stages of the disease. Fortunately, there are many breast cancer-related groups, organizations, and information on the internet, which is terrific, but it can be overwhelming trying to navigate all the links to find the "best" sites for your purposes. With the plethora of information, some of which might be inaccurate, finding accurate, appropriate evidence-based information can be a daunting task. Treatment options are rapidly evolving, as the previous chapter hopefully explained, which means keeping up with the latest evidence can be confusing. The following is provided as a reference guide and does not pretend to be a comprehensive listing by any means.

Breast Cancer Foundations and Charities

There are numerous foundations and charities dedicated to raising money for breast cancer research, providing educational information, and serving as public health advocates. In the early 1980s, for example, breast cancer advocacy initiated by newly formed foundations helped spearhead various campaigns to encourage women to perform breast self-exams, undergo mammography, and provide public education about breast cancer. In the

1990s, the pink ribbon became the symbol for breast cancer awareness, and it remains the most recognizable symbol for this disease today.

The American Cancer Society, founded in 1913 by 10 doctors and 5 lay-people in New York City, was originally called the American Society for the Control of Cancer (ASCC), and its stated mission was to educate the public about cancer. In 1936, the society formed a legion of volunteers, The Women's Field Army, whose sole purpose was to wage war on all cancer, not just breast cancer. This entity is credited with moving the organization to the forefront of voluntary health organizations. In 1945, the ASCC was reorganized and renamed the American Cancer Society (ACS), and it began raising funds to better understand cancer. Philanthropists such as Mary Lasker raised more than $4 million for the society—$1 million of which was used to establish and fund the society's groundbreaking research program. Cancer researcher, Dr. Sidney Farber, who gained fame by achieving the first clinical remission with chemotherapy ever reported for childhood leukemia, was one of the society's first research grantees. Since 1946, the ACS has invested more than $4.9 billion in research; 49 researchers funded by the society have won a Nobel Prize. Today, the scope and breadth of the ACS is multifaceted, and it remains one of the leading cancer organizations in the world. Among other things, the ACS website has links to resources and support programs in local areas of the country (https://www.cancer.org/).

The Susan G. Komen Breast Cancer Foundation was founded in 1982 in memory of Susan Komen, who died from breast cancer at the age of 36. Its mission is to end breast cancer by investing in science to find cures for the disease and to empower women with breast cancer to live with their disease. Komen affiliates have been formed across the country to support local women and raise funds. The foundation also has raised money to support community health and education programs around the world. Probably the foundation's most recognizable impact is the Komen Race for the Cure™. First held in Dallas Texas in 1983, the Komen Race for the Cure™ has grown exponentially since that time. The foundation website (https://ww5.komen .org/) states clearly and emphatically that one of its goals is "to do everything it can" to ensure that all people, especially the most vulnerable, have access to and utilize high-quality breast cancer care. As part of this mission, the foundation established the African-American Health Equity Initiative to end disparities in breast cancer outcomes in the African American community. They also hold local 3-day, 60-mile walkathons to raise money for breast cancer research. Over the past 16 years, the foundation has raised more than $848 million from these events. By funding cutting-edge research, the foundation hopes to achieve one of its goals to reduce breast cancer deaths by 50% in the United States by 2026.

The Dr. Susan Love Foundation for Breast Cancer Research was established in 1983 by Dr. Otto W. Sartorius, a breast cancer surgeon and researcher with the objective of pursuing research and promoting breast disease education. In 1995, a year after Dr. Sartorius's death, the foundation's board named Dr. Susan Love, a breast surgeon and the foundation's medical director, to lead the foundation (https://drsusanloveresearch.org/). Dr. Love was one of the "founding mothers" of the breast cancer advocacy movement in the early 1990s, being one of the founders of the National Breast Cancer Coalition (NBCC). Her best-selling book, *Dr. Susan Love's Breast Book*, fifth edition, was considered by many to be "the Bible for women with breast cancer." The foundation changed its name to the Susan Love MD Breast Cancer Research Foundation in 2000 to honor Dr. Love. The foundation's mission is to end breast cancer, and numerous research projects have been funded to achieve this aim. In 2008, the foundation set up the Army of Women, which is designed to link researchers and breast cancer survivors for breast cancer clinical studies. Specifically, the Army of Women brings together women (and men) of every ethnicity, including those with and without breast cancer and those at high risk, and breast cancer researchers. Since its inception, the Army of Women has attracted more than 376,000 volunteers willing to consider participating in research to find the cause and prevention of breast cancer.

Living beyond Breast Cancer (LBBC) was founded in 1991 by Marisa C. Weiss, MD, a radiation oncologist, who started the charity from her home with the support of local volunteers (https://www.lbbc.org/). The foundation's mission is to provide information and support to women with breast cancer after completing breast cancer treatment, as well as to offer programs that support caregivers and health care professionals. Reach & Raise raises money through community-based yoga events around the country.

The National Breast Cancer Foundation was founded in 1991 by Janelle Hail, a breast cancer survivor, to help women with breast cancer through early detection, education, and support (https://www.nationalbreastcancer.org/). The foundation provides free mammograms to women in need and also funds breast cancer education programs, awareness campaigns, and research. Game Pink is their innovative, year-round fundraiser in which online gamers can raise funds by putting their gaming skills to the test.

The NBCC, founded in 1991 by breast cancer survivors, is a grassroots advocacy organization dedicated to ending breast cancer (http://www.stopbreastcancer.org/). The NBCC links hundreds of organizations and tens of thousands of individuals into a dynamic, diverse coalition. Coalition members include breast cancer support, information, and service groups as well as women's health and provider organizations. In 1992, the NBCC was instrumental in the Department of Defense's multibillion-dollar breast cancer research project that has attracted more than 42,118 research proposals. To date, the NBCC has generated over $3.6 billion for breast cancer research. The NBCC launched the Breast Cancer Deadline 2020, a call to action for policymakers, researchers, breast cancer advocates, and other stakeholders to eradicate the disease by January 1, 2020. Since this goal was not met, the NBCC continues to strive to find a cure for breast cancer.

The Breast Cancer Research Foundation (BCRF) was founded in 1992 by Evelyn Lauder, at the time a breast cancer survivor (she died of the disease in 2011) and senior corporate vice president of Estée Lauder Companies, to help fund research and raise public awareness of the disease (https://www.bcrf .org/). Ms. Lauder was the co-creator of the original pink ribbon launched in 1992 with Alexandra Penney, former editor in chief of *Self* magazine. Since its inception, the BCRF has raised more than half a billion dollars in support of research on tumor biology, heredity and ethnicity, and lifestyle, making it one of the largest nonprofit funders of breast cancer research worldwide. The foundation also is the largest private funder of metastatic breast cancer research. The Evelyn H. Lauder Founder's Fund is a multiyear international program dedicated to metastasis. The NBCF has an online support group, Beyond the Shock, available 24-7 where one can ask questions of breast cancer survivors, learn more about breast cancer, and hear the inspiring stories of those living with breast cancer. The foundation also created a list of third-party organizations that provide in-person support groups.

The Young Survival Coalition (https://www.youngsurvival.org/) was formed in 1998 by a group of young women, all diagnosed with breast cancer before age 40. The coalition focuses on the unique needs of young adults diagnosed with breast cancer and now an international movement with 170 Face 2 Face local networking groups, which are local, in-person support groups for young women at all stages of breast cancer and in-person support groups for cosurvivors. The networks provide support and resources to empower women and to enable them to learn from each other. The coalition also has one of the largest conference programs dedicated exclusively to young adults with breast cancer and their caregivers.

Breastcancer.org is a nonprofit organization founded in 2000 by breast oncologist Dr. Marisa C. Weiss (https://www.breastcancer.org/). The organization is one of the leading patient-focused resources for breast health and breast cancer information and support. Its mission is to help people make sense of the complex medical and personal information about breast health and breast cancer to enable individuals to make educated, informed decisions about their treatment. Their website is one of the largest online breast cancer peer-to-peer community support groups, with over 226,000 registered members.

The Metastatic Breast Cancer Network (MBCN) was founded in 2004 to provide support for individuals with advanced breast cancer (http://mbcn .org/about-us/). The organization is a volunteer, patient-led advocacy organization that seeks to address the unique needs and concerns of those living with metastatic or Stage IV breast cancer. In addition to providing educational material about advanced breast cancer, the organization also advocates for research to find more targeted therapies for metastatic breast cancer.

The Pink Fund, a nonprofit organization established in 2006 by breast cancer survivor Molly MacDonald, provides financial support to help meet basic needs, allowing breast cancer patients in active treatment to focus on healing without worrying about how to pay for the treatment (https://www .pinkfund.org/). Their 90-day grant program enables breast cancer survivors to meet their expenses for housing, transportation, utilities, and insurance.

METAvivor is a nonprofit organization established by a small group of proactive metastatic breast cancer patients (https://www.metavivor.org/). METAvivor is internationally recognized for raising awareness and funds explicitly for Stage 4 breast cancer research. To highlight the need for research that is focused on advanced breast cancer, METAvivor designed a ribbon of green and teal to represent metastasis.

Support Groups

In addition to the preceding organizations, there are numerous other breast cancer patient support groups that one can find online. These groups provide a safe space for individuals to connect with others coping with breast cancer and are usually led by health care professionals with expertise in cancer care, who are trained to provide emotional and practical support. The organization CancerCare, for example, provides counseling and support services (https:// www.cancercare.org/support_groups/43-breast_cancer_patient_support _group).

Those with metastatic breast cancer have different needs from those with localized breast cancer. The Metastatic Breast Cancer Alliance (MBC Alliance) was formed in 2013 to provide information and support through various means, including MBC Connect 2.0, an interactive, free, web, and mobile-friendly patient registry. Through this portal, individuals can share information about metastatic breast cancer, personal experiences, and issues of quality of life. It was designed by patients for patients. Based on information that an individual enters, MBC Connect will send personalized insights and alerts with MBC news, events, and clinical trial opportunities (www .mbcalliance.org).

Hear My Voice Metastatic Outreach Program, part of the MBC Alliance, is designed to help individuals learn how to educate others about metastatic breast cancer and connect those living with the disease to resources and a sense of community. Hear My Voice Advocates are trained how to use their personal stories along with statistics and insights about metastatic breast cancer to increase awareness (https://www.lbbc.org/living-metastatic-breast -cancer/hear-my-voice-program/hear-my-voice-how-apply).

The Metastatic Breast Cancer Project (https://www.mbcproject.org/) is part of Count Me In, a nonprofit organization that brings together patients and researchers as partners to accelerate discoveries in cancer research (https://www.joincountmein.org/). Their goal is to perform genomics studies that will lead to understanding of the genomic underpinnings of metastatic breast cancer. Those interested in participating in this cutting-edge project sign a consent form to allow Count Me In to obtain an individual's medical records, saliva, and a portion of stored tumor samples. Their database of genomic and medical information (all de-identified to ensure confidentiality) will be shared with the National Institutes of Health and the cancer research community so as to be used for genomic and molecular studies to help understand metastatic breast cancer. Presently over 7,000 individuals have participated in this novel program. Over the next several years, Count Me In aims to enroll more than 100,000 patients living with all major cancer types, as well as rare cancers.

Facebook offers an online support community for breast cancer patients. Users can access the numerous breast cancer chat groups, most of which are private, providing a safe place to ask questions and share stories with others in a similar situation.

Breast Cancer Apps

There seems to be an app for just about anything, and breast cancer is no exception. Apparently there are over 1,000 breast cancer mobile health (mHealth) apps! Various mobile apps, available for downloading on either Android or iPhones, are designed to help you organize your treatment and ease the stress that accompanies a diagnosis of breast cancer. How effective and how helpful are mHealth apps? A systematic review of studies that scientifically tested interventions using an mHealth app specifically for breast cancer care was conducted to answer these questions.[1] A total of 29 studies, which encompassed important phases in breast cancer care and addressed prevention and survivorship, were identified. Majority of the identified studies in patients' care management showed a positive impact of the use of mHealth apps. However, the role of mHealth-based interventions in the psychological impact of treatment is less clear. Part of the problem is that only two studies addressed this topic, and neither showed convincing data on the effect of mHealth on psychological dimensions (i.e., anxiety and depression). The authors acknowledge that the effects of using mHealth breast cancer apps have not been fully studied, and of those few studies that have been published, the results are mixed. Clearly, there is a need for further study in order to draw conclusions on the utility, effectiveness, and safety of mHealth apps in breast cancer care.

While the following presents several options, I have actually not tested any of them so cannot speak personally about the pros and cons of each or endorse one over the other. Each individual has her own reasons for choosing to use an app; therefore, feel free to explore the options and select the ones that best meets your needs.

CareZone is an app that is designed to simplify medication management by keeping a list of medicines, dosages, and schedules to help you stay organized. The app also sends reminders when it's time to take a medication or to refill a prescription. The app is free of charge.

Breast Cancer Healthline, also a free app, serves to connect people with breast cancer. Those who are newly diagnosed, receiving treatment, or in remission can participate in one-on-one chats as well as group discussions. The app also provides updates on current research findings.

My Cancer Coach provides information about personalized cancer treatments (not only breast cancer) to enable the user to better manage the disease. This free app provides easy-to-understand answers to questions about breast, prostate, and colon cancer. Features include a questionnaire and personalized treatment report, questions to ask your doctor, videos and resources, a journal, a calendar, and a glossary of common terms.

Check Yourself!, designed by the Keep a Breast Foundation, is a free app that focuses on breast self-examination. The app provides instruction on doing a breast self-exam, and it lets the user set a schedule for breast self-exams and includes an automatic monthly reminder.

Pocket Cancer Care Guide includes hundreds of cancer-related questions and answers to provide information about all stages of cancer treatment. Users can create their own questions, and the app also records and stores your doctor's and nurse's answers to your questions. The app is free of charge.

Happify is a free interactive app, featuring games and guided relaxation to help the user reduce stress.

Breast Screening Decisions is a free decision aid app designed by physicians at Weill Cornell Medicine. The app provides basic information about the benefits and harms of screening mammograms for women at any age and provides a breast cancer risk assessment screening tool. Based on responses to the questions, the app calculates your chance of developing breast cancer in the next five years.

Telemedicine

Telemedicine relies on modern technology, including high-quality videoconferencing tools. During these virtual visits, the doctor and patient each sit in front of a camera and can communicate remotely. Without getting into the technicalities of this technology, telemedicine involves the use of electronic communications and software to provide clinical services to patients without an in-person visit. In order to safeguard privacy, providers must choose technology solutions that use data encryption to protect patient data.

Telemedicine technology is frequently used for follow-up visits, management of chronic conditions, and medication management, which can be provided remotely via secure video and audio connections. Private insurance plans reimburse providers for telemedicine visits, but compensation rates vary based on state legislation. Currently, Medicare reimburses providers for a telemedicine visit for office, hospital visits, and other services that generally occur in person.

The Breast Cancer Tele-Access Project at New York Presbyterian Hospital-Weill Cornell Medicine in New York is an innovative service that enables breast cancer patients to schedule a 20-minute video visit with a breast cancer access nurse to learn about cancer care at the medical center. The nurse will review the patient's medical information, answer questions, and make a referral to an appropriate specialist (i.e., radiation oncologist, breast surgeon) based on the patient's needs. Other medical centers are working to integrate telemedicine into their cancer service.

As telemedicine is increasingly being used for cancer care, any discussion of a prognosis or treatment plans needs to be done in person. Telemedicine is not a substitute for in-person care, especially when discussing sensitive, potentially upsetting issues.

What about Clinical Trials?

Many cancer patients are invited to participate in randomized clinical trials (RCTs). RCTs are considered to be the best way to assess whether a new treatment or drug is better than existing treatments or drugs. That is, the RCT is designed to test the efficacy, effectiveness, and safety of a new treatment or drug. Individuals considering participating in an RCT must be told at the outset that participation may not confer a benefit and may expose the individual to unknown risks. A "good" outcome is not guaranteed.

Every RCT must clearly state the trial's objective (i.e., what is the main objective of the trail—to compare one drug to another? One treatment to another?), eligibility requirements (i.e., age, disease, disease status), duration of the trial, trial sponsor, and name and phone number of a person or an office that you can contact for more information.

All RCTs must receive institutional review board (IRB) approval. This means that an independent group of experts (i.e., physicians, epidemiologists, biostatisticians) reviews the RCT protocol to ensure protection for human subjects in biomedical and behavioral research. In a sense, IRBs are ethical watchdogs designed to protect participants from harm. Independent review of clinical research by an IRB is required for U.S. studies funded by the Department of Health and Human Services (DHHS) and other U.S. federal agencies, as well as for research testing interventions, such as drugs, biologics, and devices, which are under the jurisdiction of the U.S. Food and Drug Administration (FDA).

The main purpose of clinical trials is to assess and evaluate a new treatment or drug in people. Individuals who participate in an RCT are known as "subjects of research" and not as patients, *per se*. Briefly, RCTs are intervention studies in which eligible participants are allocated at random (by chance alone) to either receive the clinical intervention of interest (i.e., a treatment or a drug) or to serve as the control group. The latter group does not receive the experimental treatment or drug; rather, they receive either a placebo or a treatment or drug that is currently being used as a point of comparison. In an RCT, each of the eligible participants should have an equal chance to be allocated the intervention group without interference from the physician or even from the patient. The process is random, which serves to minimize bias in treatment assignment. Bias can dilute a study's findings and weaken the value of the study.

The two groups are then followed up to see if there are any differences between them in outcome. Statistical analysis of the data serves to assess the effectiveness of the intervention. RCTs are the most stringent way of determining whether a cause-effect relation exists between the intervention and the outcome. Most RCTs are double blinded studies, which means that neither the physician nor the patient knows whether the patient will receive the experimental treatment or drug or not. The treatment assignment is not known in advance to either the physician or the patient. This also reduces the possibility of bias, which refers to the deviation of results from the truth, due to systematic error in the research methodology.

In order for an RCT to be scientifically valid, the comparison between groups depends on the groups being alike as much as possible, with the only exception being the specific treatments under investigation. If the groups differ on key factors (i.e., age, gender, disease stage) at the outset, the integrity of the study would be compromised. It would be like comparing apples to oranges, and one would not be able to state with statistical certainty that the intervention was statistically "better" than that to which it was being compared. Table 1 of any RCT is one of the most important pieces of information, as it describes the characteristics of the experimental group and the control group. If there are statistically significant differences between the groups, the value of the study is weakened. Restriction of the study to a specific group of relatively homogeneous patients can nearly always minimize potential differences in the study population and thus minimize potential bias.

Another important caveat of an RCT is that the duration of the study must be sufficiently long enough for participants to reach the stated endpoint (i.e., survival, improvements in quality of life, relief of symptoms, disappearance of the tumor). If, for example, it is known that a specific drug will take six weeks to have some effect, the RCT has to last much longer than six weeks in order to see any potential differences among the participants.

Not every participant will remain in the study until the end of the trial. In some cases the burdens or side effects of participating in the trial may be too much to bear, prompting some people to drop out before the end of the study. Withdrawal from the study and loss to follow-up are both factors that can negatively impact the study's findings. How the researchers account for withdrawal and loss to follow-up must be clearly described in the final report. A good rule of thumb is that less than a 5% loss of participants is acceptable, while greater than 20% poses serious threats to the validity of the study.

Before a physician raises the possibility of the patient participating in an RCT, the physician must determine the extent to which the RCT will be potentially beneficial to the patient. The potential risks and benefits of participating in the RCT must be explained clearly so that the patient can make an informed decision. For all intents and purposes, the risks must not outweigh the benefits. For this reason, a clear, easily understandable informed consent policy for RCTs is essential.

Every RCT must include in its protocol Informed consent. This is an ethical and legal prerequisite for trial participation. Prospective participants must be informed (orally and in writing) about the purpose of the trial, what will be done to them, expected length of time for participation, what risks or discomforts they may experience, and what potential benefits may be gained. By convention, informed consent must be very detailed in scope and content, including adequate information to allow for an informed decision about participation in the clinical investigation in a way that the individual can understand, an acknowledgment that participation is voluntary. There must be sufficient opportunity for the participant to consider whether to participate or not. Individuals should not feel pressured to participate. There must be an acknowledgment that the participant may not benefit from the clinical trial and may be exposed to unknown risks. Importantly, it must be clearly stated that individuals may drop out of the study at any time.

The informed consent form also must have a statement describing how confidentiality of information collected during the clinical trial will be ensured. Identified and de-identified records must be handled differently. RCTs assign unique ID numbers rather than have the individual's name on forms (i.e., de-identified data), but for those records that list identifying information (i.e., name of patient), there must be a plan in place to ensure confidentiality (i.e., how will these records be stored?).

The National Cancer Institute (NCI) has an excellent website describing the nature and purpose of RCTs, including the types and phases of trials and how they are carried out (https://www.cancer.gov/about-cancer/treatment /clinical-trials/what-are-trials). The NCI also provides information on how to find a clinical trial; however, the best first step is to talk to your doctor about options. Some trials may not be appropriate for you! (See https://www.cancer .gov/about-cancer/treatment/clinical-trials/search/trial-guide.) The NCI network trials website lists NCI-supported clinical trials that are taking place across the United States, Canada, and internationally, including trials supported through the National Clinical Trials Network (NCTN), NCI Community Oncology Research Program (NCORP), and Experimental Therapeutics Clinical Trials Network (ETCTN) and trials taking place at NCI-Designated Cancer Centers.[2] More information can be obtained by calling the NCI's Cancer Information Service (1-800-4-CANCER [1-800-422-6237]).

It is important to realize that there are many lists and sponsors of cancer clinical trials. Trials are funded by nonprofit organizations, the federal government, and drug companies. Hospitals and academic medical centers also sponsor trials conducted by their own researchers. No one list should be considered to be the most comprehensive. It depends on who made the list and which trials are included in that list. RCTs take place in many different locations, some of which may be near to where you live. The protocol for each trial should explain the goal of the trial, which treatments will be tested, and the location where the trial is taking place.

Other resources include the following:

- ClinicalTrials.gov, which is part of the National Library of Medicine, lists clinical trials for cancer and many other diseases and conditions. This site also lists trials sponsored by pharmaceutical or biotech companies that may not be on NCI's list.

- Many cancer centers across the United States, including NCI-Designated Cancer Centers, sponsor or take part in cancer clinical trials. The websites of these centers (i.e., Memorial Sloan Kettering Cancer Center) usually have a list of the clinical trials taking place at their institutions. Some of the trials included in these lists may not be on NCI's list.

- The Pharmaceutical Research and Manufacturers of America (PhRMA), a trade organization that represents drug and biotechnology companies in the United States, includes a list of its member companies, many of which sponsor cancer clinical trials.

There are organizations that focus on RCTs for specific cancers. For example, BreastCancerTrials.org helps individuals diagnosed with breast cancer find "the trial that is right for you" (https://www.breastcancertrials.org/BCTIncludes /index.html;jsessionid=kqxTnzJRG4eH1yQHCgnruJyY_RKXTZ6YW5D9 Jn9h.ip-10-20-10-73). It should be noted that in breast cancer trials, no group will be given a placebo. Participants will either be given standard of care (the best treatment available for their specific cancer) or receive a new treatment that is being investigated. Placebos are never used when a breast cancer patient would be put at risk by not having effective therapy for their cancer.

You Are Not Alone

Perhaps the toughest thing that happens when you receive a breast cancer diagnosis is that you feel all alone. My mother, upon hearing that she was diagnosed with breast cancer at age 53, questioned, "Why me?" Hopefully the information in this chapter shows that no patient should feel that she is alone in her fight against cancer. Every breast cancer patient has a team of medical professionals who are focused on providing the best course of treatment *for you*. Every breast cancer patient has unique needs, and the team is there to advise and guide you as you undergo treatment and thereafter. There are so many help groups, websites for information, and organizations whose mission is to make the ordeal of cancer treatment easier for the individual. Clinical trials are being conducted to help find if not a cure for cancer then a means of treating the cancer so that the individual can have a somewhat normal life while living with her cancer. There are so many opportunities to reach out for help, advice, and support. All one has to do is ask!

Appendix: Breast Cancer Screening Guidelines for Women

	U.S. Preventive Services Task Force (2016)[1]	American Cancer Society (2015)[2]	American College of Obstetricians and Gynecologists (2011)[3]	International Agency for Research on Cancer (2015)[4]	American College of Radiology (2010)[5]	American College of Physicians (2015)[6]	American Academy of Family Physicians (2016)[7]
Women aged 40–49 with average risk	The decision to start screening mammography in women prior to age 50 years should be an individual one. Women who place a higher value on the potential benefit than the potential harms may choose to begin biennial screening between the ages of 40 and 49 years.	*Women aged 40–44 years* should have the choice to start annual breast cancer screening with mammograms if they wish to do so. The risks of screening as well as the potential benefits should be considered. *Women aged 45–49 years* should get mammograms every year.	Screening with mammography and clinical breast exams annually.	Insufficient evidence to recommend for or against screening.	Screening with mammography annually.	Discuss benefits and harms with women in good health and order screening with mammography every two years if a woman requests it.	The decision to start screening mammography should be an individual one. Women who place a higher value on the potential benefit than the potential harms may choose to begin screening.

Women aged 50–74 with average risk	Biennial screening mammography is recommended.	Women aged 50–54 years should get mammograms every year. Women aged 55 years and older should switch to mammograms every two years or have the choice to continue yearly screening.	Screening with mammography and clinical breast exam annually.	For women aged 50–69 years, screening with mammography is recommended. For women aged 70–74 years, evidence suggests that screening with mammography substantially reduces the risk of death from breast cancer, but it is not currently recommended.	Screening with mammography annually.	Physicians should encourage mammography screening every two years in average-risk women.	Biennial screening with mammography.

(continued)

	U.S. Preventive Services Task Force (2016)	American Cancer Society (2015)	American College of Obstetricians and Gynecologists (2011)	International Agency for Research on Cancer (2015)	American College of Radiology (2010)	American College of Physicians (2015)	American Academy of Family Physicians (2016)
Women aged 75 or older with average risk	Current evidence is insufficient to assess the balance of benefits and harms of screening mammography in women aged 75 years or older.	Screening should continue as long as a woman is in good health and is expected to live 10 more years or longer.	Women should, in consultation with their physicians, decide whether or not to continue mammographic screening.	Not addressed.	Screening with mammography should stop when life expectancy is less than 5–7 years on the basis of age or comorbid conditions.	Screening is not recommended.	Current evidence is insufficient to assess the balance of benefits and harms of screening with mammography.
Women with dense breasts	Current evidence is insufficient to assess the balance of benefits and harms of adjunctive screening for breast cancer using breast	There is not enough evidence to make a recommendation for or against yearly MRI screening.	Insufficient evidence to recommend for or against MRI screening.	Insufficient evidence to recommend for or against screening.	In addition to mammography, ultrasound can be considered.	Not addressed.	Current evidence is insufficient to assess the balance of benefits and harms of adjunctive screening for breast cancer

ultrasonography, magnetic resonance imaging (MRI), digital breast tomosynthesis (DBT), or other methods in women identified to have dense breasts on an otherwise negative screening mammogram.

using breast ultrasonography, MRI, DBT, or other methods.

(continued)

	U.S. Preventive Services Task Force (2016)	American Cancer Society (2015)	American College of Obstetricians and Gynecologists (2011)	International Agency for Research on Cancer (2015)	American College of Radiology (2010)	American College of Physicians (2015)	American Academy of Family Physicians (2016)
Women at higher-than-average risk	Women with a parent, sibling, or child with breast cancer are at higher risk for breast cancer and thus may benefit more than average-risk women from beginning screening in their 40s.	Women who are at high risk for breast cancer based on certain factors (such as having a parent, sibling, or child with a *BRCA1* or *BRCA2* gene mutation) should get an MRI and a mammogram every year.	*For women who test positive for BRCA1 or BRCA2 mutations or have a lifetime risk of 20% or greater, screening should include twice-yearly clinical breast exams, annual mammography, annual breast MRI, and breast self-exams.*	Evidence suggests that screening (mammography and MRI) at an earlier age may be beneficial.	*For BRCA1 or BRCA2 mutation carriers, untested family members of BRCA1 or BRCA2 mutation carriers, and women with a lifetime risk of 20% or greater (based on family history), screening should include annual mammography and annual MRI starting by age 30 years but not before age 25 years.*	Not addressed.	Not addressed.

For women who received thoracic irradiation between ages 10 and 30 years, screening should include annual mammography, annual MRI, and screening clinical breast exams every 6–12 months beginning 8–10 years after radiation treatment or at age 25 years.

For women with a history of chest irradiation between the ages of 10 and 30 years, annual mammography and annual MRI should start 8 years after treatment (mammography not recommended before age 25).

(continued)

	U.S. Preventive Services Task Force (2016)	American Cancer Society (2015)	American College of Obstetricians and Gynecologists (2011)	International Agency for Research on Cancer (2015)	American College of Radiology (2010)	American College of Physicians (2015)	American Academy of Family Physicians (2016)
Additional issues relevant for all women	Current evidence is insufficient to assess the benefits and harms of digital breast Tomosynthesis (DBT) as a primary screening method for breast cancer.	Women should be familiar with the known benefits, limitations, and potential harms associated with breast cancer screening. They should also be familiar with how their breasts normally look and feel and report any changes to a health care provider right away.	Not addressed.	Not addressed.	Not addressed.	Annual mammography, MRI, tomosynthesis, or regular systematic breast self-exam are not recommended.	Recommends against clinicians teaching women breast self-exams. Current evidence is insufficient to assess the benefits and harms of clinical breast exams and DBT.

[1]Siu AL; U.S. Preventive Services Task Force. Screening for breast cancer: U.S. Preventive Services Task Force recommendation statement. *Ann Intern Med.* 2016; 164(4): 279–296.

[2]Oeffinger KC, Fontham ET, Etzioni R, et al. Breast cancer screening for women at average risk: 2015 guideline update from the American Cancer Society. *JAMA.* 2015; 314(15): 1599–1614.

[3]American College of Obstetricians-Gynecologists. Practice bulletin no. 122: Breast cancer screening. *Obstet Gynecol.* 2011; 118(2 Pt 1): 372–382.

[4]Lauby-Secretan B, Loomis D, Straif K. Breast-cancer screening—viewpoint of the IARC Working Group. *N Engl J Med.* 2015; 373(15): 1478–1479.

[5]Lee CH, Dershaw DD, Kopans D, et al. Breast cancer screening with imaging: recommendations from the Society of Breast Imaging and the ACR on the use of mammography, breast MRI, breast ultrasound, and other technologies for the detection of clinically occult breast cancer. *J Am Coll Radiol.* 2010; 7(1): 18–27.

[6]Wilt TJ, Harris RP, Qaseem A; High Value Care Task Force of the American College of Physicians. Screening for cancer: advice for high-value care from the American College of Physicians. *Ann Intern Med.* 2015; 162(10): 718–725.

[7]American Academy of Family Physicians. Summary of Recommendations for Clinical Preventive Services. 2016. http://www.aafp.org/dam/AAFP/documents/patient_care/clinical_recommendations/cps-recommendations.pdf [PDF-574KB] (Date accessed April 30, 2020).

Glossary

Adenosis: A condition when some of the lobules (milk-producing sacs) grow larger and contain more glands than usual and can cause breast pain. Adenosis does not increase the risk of breast cancer, but a biopsy is needed to tell the difference between adenosis and cancer.

Adjuvant Therapy: A cancer treatment method used in addition to (adjuvant to) surgery, radiation, chemotherapy, or hormone therapy.

Aromatase Inhibitors (AIs): A type of adjuvant treatment that works by blocking the enzyme aromatase, the enzyme that converts androgens into estrogen, thus limiting the supply of estrogen that helps promote the growth of some breast cancers.

Atypia: Structural abnormality in a cell, but atypical cells aren't necessarily cancerous.

Axillary Lymph Node Dissection: Surgery to remove some of the lymph nodes in the armpit.

Axillary Node: One of the lymph glands of the axilla (armpit) that helps to fight infections in the chest, armpit, neck, and arm and to drain lymph from those areas.

Benign: A noncancerous growth.

Biological (Immunological) Targeted Therapy: A type of adjuvant treatment that uses living organisms, substances derived from organisms, or laboratory-made versions of those substances to stimulate the body's immune system to act against cancer cells. Tailored or targeted therapy based on the presence or absence of receptors for estrogen, progesterone, and HER2 is the basis for biological targeted therapy.

Biopsy: The removal and microscopic examination of tissue for diagnosis. A biopsy can be done surgically or with needles.

BRCA1: A gene that, when mutated, increases the risk of breast, ovarian, pancreatic, cervical, uterine, and colon cancers. *BRCA1* mutations are also associated with an increased risk of triple-negative breast cancer, an aggressive and frequently difficult to treat cancer.

BRCA2: A gene that, when mutated, increases the risk of breast, ovarian, pancreatic, gallbladder, bile duct, and melanoma cancers.

Brachytherapy: The use of radioactive material in the form of a seed, pellet, wire, or capsule that is implanted in the body using a needle or catheter.

Breast-Conserving Surgery: A surgery that removes only the tumor and small amount of surrounding breast tissue (e.g., lumpectomy).

Breast Ducts: Passageways that carry milk from the lobules to the nipple.

Breast Lobules: Glandular tissue that contains cells that make and secrete milk.

Breast Reconstruction: A surgical procedure using autologous tissue (a person's own skin and tissues), implants, or both either at the time of the mastectomy or thereafter. Breast reconstruction also can be done many months or even years after breast surgery.

Breast Self-Exam: Physical examination of the breasts by the woman to detect lumps or other unusual signs of breast disease.

Cancer: A group of diseases in which cells are changed (mutated) in appearance and function and grow out of control.

Chemotherapy: A type of adjuvant treatment that is designed to kill or damage cancer cells. These agents are given intravenously or orally, and usually multiple combinations of drugs can be used.

Clinical Breast Exam: Physical examination of the breasts by a physician or trained health professional with the intent of finding lumps or other unusual signs of breast disease.

Clinical Outcome: End result of a medical intervention (e.g., survival, improved health, death).

Clinical Trial: A study intended to quantify the safety or effectiveness of a drug, procedure, or medical intervention. Clinical trials can be randomized or non-randomized. (See Randomized Clinical Trial.)

Digital Infrared Imaging/Breast Thermography: Detects the heat produced by increased blood vessel circulation based on images of temperature variations, which can signify very early signs of breast cancer or precancer.

Digital Mammography/Digital Breast Tomosynthesis: A type of mammography that can detect tumors not visible on mammography. Whereas screen-film mammography uses x-ray equipment to record images, digital mammography uses more specialized computerized equipment to capture a digital image and delivers lower doses of radiation. It improves detection of tumors in women with dense breasts.

Ductal Carcinoma In Situ (DCIS): Also called intraductal carcinoma. Is an early, noninvasive or preinvasive form of breast cancer.

Dysplasia: Abnormal change in cells leading to abnormal growth.

Effectiveness: The extent to which a specific test or intervention does what it is intended to do.

Epidemiology: The science of quantifying the distribution and determinants of disease in populations.

Estrogen: A hormone essential for the normal growth and development of the breast. The main forms of estrogen in females (endogenous estrogen) include estradiol, the main estrogen made by the ovaries before menopause; estrone, a weaker estrogen produced in the ovaries and in fat tissue from other hormones; and estriol, produced almost exclusively during pregnancy.

Estrogen Positive: Cancer cells grow in response to the estrogen hormone.

False Negative Test: A test result that indicates that an abnormality or disease is not present when in fact it is.

False Positive Test: A test result that indicates that an abnormality or disease is present when in fact it is not.

Fibroadenomas: Painless round or oval, firm, rubbery in consistency lumps of the breast tissue that arise from an excess growth of glandular and connective tissues. They are the most common type of benign breast tumor, and most do not increase the risk of breast cancer.

Fibrocystic Breast Disease: A benign (noncancerous) condition characterized by lumpy, nodular breasts that may cause breast pain. Fibrocystic breast changes, common throughout the menstrual cycle, do not increase the risk of breast cancer.

Genetic Screening: The means of identifying individuals who are at risk for a genetic disease or for transmitting a gene for a genetic disease. The results of a genetic test can confirm or rule out a suspected genetic condition or help determine a person's chance of developing or passing on a genetic disorder.

HER2-Positive Breast Cancer: A breast cancer that tests positive for a protein called human epidermal growth factor receptor 2 (HER2), which promotes the growth of cancer cells. The cancer cells have a gene mutation that makes an excess of the HER2 protein.

Hormonal-Receptor Negative (HR–): Cancer cells that are estrogen receptor negative do not need estrogen to grow and usually do not stop growing when treated with hormones that block estrogen from binding.

Hormonal-Receptor Positive (HR+): Cancer cells that are estrogen receptor positive have receptors for the hormones estrogen or progesterone. These cells need estrogen or progesterone to grow.

Hormonal Therapy/Endocrine Therapy: An adjuvant treatment designed to control the growth of hormone receptor positive breast cancer cells by blocking the receptors, lowering the hormone levels, or eliminating receptors.

Hormone Therapy: A type of adjuvant treatment in which drugs are used to slow tumor growth by blocking the effect of certain hormones. This therapy is designed to prevent cancer recurrence.

Hyperplasia: An overgrowth of the cells that line the ducts or the milk glands. There are two types of hyperplasia: ductal hyperplasia (also called duct epithelial hyperplasia) or lobular hyperplasia. Hyperplasia can increase the risk of breast cancer.

Incidence: The number of new cases of disease in a population at a specific period of time (e.g., a year).

Invasive Cancer: Cancerous tumors that have grown beyond their site of origin and have invaded surrounding tissue.

Invasive Ductal Carcinoma: Sometimes called infiltrating ductal carcinoma. The cancer originates in the milk ducts, but unlike DCIS, the cancer has "invaded" or spread to the surrounding breast tissues.

Invasive Lobular Carcinoma: A cancer that originates in the milk-producing glands (lobules) of the breast and spreads to the surrounding tissue.

Lead Time Bias: The length of time between the detection of a disease and its clinical presentation and diagnosis. It is the time between early diagnosis with screening and the time in which diagnosis would have been made without screening.

Length Time Bias: Less aggressive cancers grow slower; therefore, the length of time that a cancer is detectable by screening is greater for the slow-growing tumors, leading to the perception that screening leads to better outcomes when in reality it has no effect.

Lobular Carcinoma In Situ: A benign growth change in cells lining the lobules of the milk ducts.

Lump: Any kind of mass in the breast or other parts of the body.

Lumpectomy: A surgical procedure that removes a small amount of tissue from the breast and some of the normal tissue surrounding it but not the entire breast.

Lymphedema: Swelling of the arm caused by malfunctioning lymphatic drainage. Usually occurs on the side of the body where the mastectomy or axillary dissection is performed.

Lymph Nodes: Part of the lymphatic system that helps fight infection.

Magnetic Resonance Imagining (MRI): Uses radio waves and strong magnets to create very detailed, cross-sectional 3D images of the breast. MRI of the breast can be effective for women with dense breasts, for women with breast implants (e.g., to detect leaks or ruptures), and can be used after breast cancer is detected by other means to determine the extent of the tumor.

Malignancy: A cancerous tumor.

Mammography/Mammogram: X-ray image of the breast. It is designed to show tumors in the breast before they can be felt.

Mastectomy: Surgical removal of the breast.

Metastasis: Spread of a cancer from one part of the body to another.

Microcalcifications: Tiny calcium deposits within the breast often found by mammography. They may be a sign of cancer.

Modified Radical Mastectomy: A surgical procedure in which the entire breast, including the breast tissue, skin, areola, and nipple and most of the underarm (axillary) lymph nodes, is removed, but both the pectoralis major and the pectoralis minor muscles are preserved.

Molecular Markers: Changes in cells at the molecular level.

Mutation: A change in the character of a gene that is perpetuated in subsequent divisions of the cell in which it occurs.

Negative Predictive Value: The probability that subjects with a positive screening test truly have the disease.

Nipple-Sparing Mastectomy: A variation of the skin-sparing mastectomy in which the breast tissue is removed, but the breast skin and nipple are left in place.

Oncogene: The gene that contributes to the development of a malignant tumor.

Oncologist: A physician who specializes in the treatment of cancer.

Overdiagnosis/Overdetection: The detection of cancers that grow so slowly that they are unlikely to be diagnosed during a person's lifetime and would not cause the individual any harm in the absence of screening.

Partial Mastectomy: Surgical removal of part of the breast.

Positive Predictive Value: The probability that subjects with a positive screening test truly have the disease.

Precancer: Changes in cells that may precede the development of a malignant tumor.

Prevalence: The number of existing cases of disease in a population at a specified time period (e.g., a year).

Progesterone Positive: Cancer cells grow in response to progesterone.

Prognosis: Prediction of the course of the disease and the estimated chance for recovery or survival.

Radiation Therapy: Treatment for breast cancer that uses high-energy rays to kill cancer cells. Radiation therapy treatment aims to kill, shrink, or slow the growth of cancer cells.

Radical Mastectomy: A surgical procedure in which the entire breast as well as the underlying chest muscle (including pectoralis major and pectoralis minor) and lymph nodes of the axilla is removed.

Randomized Clinical Trial: The type of study in which subjects are randomly assigned to treatment group or control/placebo group.

Recurrence: Reappearance of a cancer. Recurrence can be local (at the same site), regional (near the original site), or distant (far from the original site).

Remission: Absence of signs of cancer in the body.

Screening: Testing in an asymptomatic population with the goal of detecting a specific disease at an early stage. A screening test is designed to identify those who may have a disease and should be referred for further workup.

Selective Estrogen Receptor Modulators (SERMs): Agents that function as estrogen agonists in the tissues in which estrogen is beneficial but will function as estrogen antagonists in sites where estrogen may promote cancer.

Sensitivity: The proportion of truly diseased cases in a screened population who are identified as diseased by the screening test (e.g., true positive rate).

Simple Mastectomy: A surgical procedure in which the breast is removed, but neither the pectoralis muscles nor the axillary lymph nodes are removed.

Skin-Sparing Mastectomy: A surgical procedure in which the surgeon removes only the skin of the nipple, areola, the original biopsy scar, and the breast tissue through the small opening that is created.

Specificity: The proportion of truly nondiseased cases in a screened population who are identified as not having the disease by the screening test (e.g., true negative rate).

Surveillance, Epidemiology, and End Results (SEER) Cancer Registry: An epidemiologic surveillance system consisting of population-based tumor registries designated to track cancer incidence and survival in geographically defined areas in the United States.

Triple-Negative Breast Cancer (TNBC): Estrogen, progesterone, and the *HER-2/neu* gene are not present in the cancer. Triple-negative tumors can be aggressive and have a poorer survival rate than other types of tumors.

Tumor: An abnormal mass of tissue that results from excessive cell division. Tumors can be benign or malignant.

Tumor Marker: Any substance or characteristic that indicates the presence of a malignancy.

Ultrasound: A radiologic test that uses sound waves to create an image inside the body.

U.S. Preventive Services Taskforce: An independent, volunteer panel of national experts in disease prevention and evidence-based medicine, which makes evidence-based recommendations about clinical preventive services, including screening for disease.

Notes

Chapter 1

1. Yalom M. *A History of the Breast*. New York: Ballantine Books, 1998.

2. Ibid.

3. Ibid.

4. "brassière." The Oxford Companion to the Body. https://www.encyclopedia.com (Date accessed July 20, 2019).

5. Ibid.

6. History of Bras. https://en.wikipedia.org/wiki/History_of_bras (Date accessed July 18, 2019).

7. Benign Breast Problems and Conditions. https://www.acog.org/patient-resources/faqs/gynecologic-problems/benign-breast-problems-and-conditions (Date accessed July 18, 2019).

8. American Cancer Society. Non-cancerous Breast Conditions. https://www.cancer.org/cancer/breast-cancer/non-cancerous-breast-conditions.html (Date accessed July 18, 2019).

9. American Cancer Society. Types of Breast Cancer. https://www.cancer.org/cancer/breast-cancer/understanding-a-breast-cancer-diagnosis/types-of-breast-cancer.html (Date accessed July 18, 2019).

10. Kerlikowske K. Epidemiology of ductal carcinoma in situ. *J Natl Cancer Inst Monogr.* 2010; 2010(41): 139–141.

11. Narod SA, Iqbal J, Giannakeas V, et al. Breast cancer mortality after a diagnosis of ductal carcinoma in situ. *JAMA Oncol.* 2015; 1: 888–896.

12. American Cancer Society. Treatment of Ductal Carcinoma in Situ (DCIS). https://www.cancer.org/cancer/breast-cancer/treatment/treatment-of-breast-cancer-by-stage/treatment-of-ductal-carcinoma-in-situ-dcis.html (Date accessed July 20, 2019).

13. Narod SA and Rakovitch E. A comparison of the risks of in-breast recurrence after a diagnosis of DCIS or early invasive breast cancer. *Curr Oncol.* 2014; 21(3): 119–124.

14. Virnig BA, Wang SY, Shamilyan T, et al. Ductal carcinoma in situ: Risk factors and impact of screening. *J Natl Cancer Inst Monogr.* 2010; 2010(41): 113–116.

15. IDC Type: Medullary Carcinoma of the Breast. https://www.breastcancer .org/symptoms/types/medullary (Date accessed July 20, 2019).

16. IDC Type: Mucinous Carcinoma of the Breast. https://www.breastcancer .org/symptoms/types/mucinous (Date accessed July 20, 2019).

17. IDC Type: Tubular Carcinoma of the Breast. https://www.breastcancer.org /symptoms/types/tubular (Date accessed July 20, 2019).

18. Invasive Lobular Carcinoma (ILC). https://www.breastcancer.org/symptoms /types/ilc (Date accessed July 20, 2019).

19. History of Breast Cancer. https://www.healthline.com/health/history -of-breast-cancer (Date accessed July 20, 2019).

20. Bianucci R, Perciaccante AN, Charlier P, et al. Earliest evidence of malignant breast cancer in Renaissance paintings. *Lancet: Oncol.* 2018; 19(2): 166–167.

21. Zurrida S, Bassi F, Arnone, et al. The changing face of mastectomy (from mutilation to aid to breast reconstruction). *Int J Surg Oncol.* 2011; e2011, Article ID 980158, 7 pages. https://doi.org/10.1155/2011/980158.

Chapter 2

1. U.S. Breast Cancer Statistics. https://www.breastcancer.org/symptoms /understand_bc/statistics (Date accessed July 24, 2019).

2. Ibid.

3. Ibid.

4. World Health Organization. Preventing Cancer. https://www.who.int /cancer/prevention/diagnosis-screening/breast-cancer/en/ (Date accessed July 24, 2019).

5. National Cancer Institute. Surveillance, Epidemiology, and End Results (SEER) Program. SEER 9 Registries. https://seer.cancer.gov/ (Date accessed July 24, 2019).

6. Coombs NJ, Cronin KA, Taylor RJ, et al. The impact of changes in hormone therapy on breast cancer incidence in the US population cancer causes control. *Cancer Causes Control.* 2010; 21: 83–90.

7. American Cancer Society. Cancer Facts and Figures 2019. https://www .cancer.org/cancer/breast-cancer/about/how-common-is-breast-cancer.html (Date accessed July 24, 2019).

8. Ibid.

9. National Cancer Institute. Surveillance, epidemiology, and End Results Program (SEER). Cancer Stat Facts: Female Breast Cancer. https://seer.cancer.gov /statfacts/html/breast.html (Date accessed July 24, 2019).

10. U.S. Breast Cancer Statistics, https://www.breastcancer.org/symptoms /understand_bc/statistics.

11. Risk of Developing Breast Cancer. https://www.breastcancer.org/symptoms/understand_bc/risk/understanding (Date accessed July 26, 2019).

12. American Cancer Society. *Breast Cancer Facts and Figures 2017–2018.* Atlanta, GA: American Cancer Society, 2017.

13. Anders CK, Fan C, Parker JS, et al. Breast carcinomas arising at a young age: Unique biology or a surrogate for aggressive intrinsic subtypes? *J Clin Oncol.* 2011; 29(1): e18–e20.

14. Anders CK, Johnson R, Litton J, et al. Breast cancer before age 40 years. *Semin Oncol.* 2009; 36(3): 237–249.

15. Freedman RA and Partridge AH. Emerging data and current challenges for young, old, obese, or male patients with breast cancer. *Clin Cancer Res.* 2017; 23: 2647–2654.

16. Li CI, Malone KE, Daling JR. Differences in breast cancer stage, treatment, and survival by race and ethnicity. *Arch Int Med.* 2003; 163: 49–56.

17. American Cancer Society, https://www.cancer.org/cancer/breast-cancer/about/how-common-is-breast-cancer.html.

18. Anders et al. Breast cancer before age 40 years.

19. Bradley CJ, Given CW, Roberts C. Race, socioeconomic status, and breast cancer treatment and survival. *J Nat Cancer Inst.* 2002; 94: 490–496.

20. Collaborative Group on Hormonal Factors in Breast Cancer. Familial breast cancer: Collaborative reanalysis of individual data from 52 epidemiological studies including 58 209 women with breast cancer and 101 986 women without the disease. *Lancet.* 2001; 358: 1389–1399.

21. Lalloo F, Varley J, Moran A, et al. BRCA1 and BRCA2 and TP53 mutations in very early-onset breast cancer with associated risks to relatives. *Eur J Cancer.* 2006; 42: 1143–1150.

22. Michailidou K, Beesley J, Lindstrom S, et al. Genome-wide association analysis of more than 120,000 individuals identifies 15 new susceptibility loci for breast cancer. *Nat Genet.* 2015; 47: 373–380.

23. Primary Information of p53 gene. http://www.bioinformatics.org/p53/introduction.html (Date accessed July 30, 2019).

24. Collaborative Group on Hormonal Factors in Breast Cancer, Familial breast cancer

25. http://www.advancedbreastcancercommunity.org/pdf/asset-library/Know_Your_Type.pdf (Date accessed July 30, 2019).

26. Shimelis H, LaDuca H, Hu C, et al. Triple-negative breast cancer risk genes identified by multigene hereditary cancer panel testing. *J Natl Cancer Inst.* 2018; 110(8): 855–862.

27. Bassuk SS and Manson JE. Oral contraceptives and menopausal hormone therapy: Relative and attributable risks of cardiovascular disease, cancer, and other health outcomes. *Ann Epidemiol.* 2015; 25: 193–200.

28. Herbst AL, Ulfelder H, Poskanzer DC. Adenocarcinoma of the vagina. Association of maternal stilbestrol therapy with tumor appearance in young women. *New Engl J Med.* 1971; 284(15): 878–881.

29. Malone KE. Diethylstilbestrol (DES) and breast cancer. *Epidemiol Rev.* 1993; 15: 108–109.

30. Verloop J, van Leeuwen FE, Helmerhorst TJ, et al. Cancer risk in DES daughters. *Cancer Causes and Control.* 2010; 21(7): 999–1007.

31. Hoover RN, Hyer M, Pfeiffer RM, et al. Adverse health outcomes in women exposed in utero to diethylstilbestrol. *New Engl J Med.* 2011; 365(14): 1304–1314.

32. Salhab M, Al Sarakbi W, Mokbel K. In vitro fertilization and breast cancer risk: A review. *Int J Fertil Womens Med.* 2005; 50(6): 259–266.

33. Van den Belt-Dusebout AW, Spaan M, Lambalk CB, et al. Ovarian stimulation for in vitro fertilization and long-term risk of breast cancer. *JAMA.* 2016; 316(3): 300–312.

34. Thomson CA, McCullough ML, Wertheim BC, et al. Nutrition and physical activity cancer prevention guidelines, cancer risk, and mortality in the women's health initiative. *Cancer Prev Res (Phila).* 2014; 7(1): 42–53.

35. Baer HJ, Colditz GA, Rosner B, et al. Body fatness during childhood and adolescence and incidence of breast cancer in premenopausal women: A prospective cohort study. *Breast Cancer Res.* 2005; 7(3): R314–R325.

36. Bernstein L. Epidemiology of endocrine-related risk factors for breast cancer. *J Mammary Gland Biol Neoplasia.* 2002; 7: 3–15.

37. Keum N, Greenwood DC, Lee DH, et al. Adult weight gain and adiposity-related cancers: A dose-response meta-analysis of prospective observational studies. *J Natl Cancer Inst.* 2015; 107(2). https://doi.org/10.1093/jnci/djv088.

38. Albuquerque RC, Baltar VT, Marchioni DM. Breast cancer and dietary patterns: A systematic review. *Nutr Rev.* 2014; 72: 1–17.

39. Farvid MS, Stern MC, Norat T, et al. Consumption of red and processed meat and breast cancer incidence: A systematic review and meta-analysis of prospective studies. *Int. J Cancer.* 2018; 143(11):2787–2799.

40. US Department of Health and Human Services. *The Health Consequences of Smoking—50 Years of Progress. A report of the Surgeon General.* Atlanta, GA: Centers for Disease Control and Prevention, National Center for Chronic Disease Prevention and Health Promotion, Office on Smoking and Health, 2014.

41. Gaudet MM, Gapstur SM, Sun J, et al. Active smoking and breast cancer risk: Original cohort data and meta-analysis. *J Natl Cancer Inst.* 2013; 105: 515–525.

42. Hildebrand JS, Gapstur SM, Campbell PT, et al. Recreational physical activity and leisure-time sitting in relation to postmenopausal breast cancer risk. *Cancer Epidemiol Biomarkers Prev.* 2013; 22: 1906–1912.

43. Anstey EH, Shoemaker ML, Barrera CH, et al. Breastfeeding and breast cancer risk reduction: Implications for Black mothers. *Am J Prev Med.* 2017; 53(3 Suppl 1): S40–S46.

44. FDA Says Mammography Reports Should Provide More Information on Breast Density. https://www.breastcancer.org/research-news/fda-says-mammos-need-more-density-info (Date accessed July 30, 2019).

45. Sabel MS. Overview of Benign Breast Disease. https://www.uptodate.com /contents/overview-of-benign-breast-disease (Date accessed July 31, 2019).

46. Clemens MW and Miranda RN. Coming of age: Breast implant-associated anaplastic large cell lymphoma after 18 years of investigation. *Clin Plastic Surg.* 2015; 42: 605–613.

47. Collaborative Group on Hormonal Factors in Breast Cancer. Breast cancer and breastfeeding: Collaborative reanalysis of individual data from 47 epidemiological studies in 30 countries, including 50302 women with breast cancer and 96973 women without the disease. *Lancet.* 2002; 360(9328): 187–195.

48. Gammon MD, Neugut Aim Santella RM, et al. The Long Island Breast Cancer Study Project: Description of a multi-institutional collaboration to identify environmental risk factors for breast cancer. *Brest Cancer Res Treat.* 2002; 74: 235–254.

49. Schoenfeld ER, O'Leary ES, Henderson K, et al. Electromagnetic fields and breast cancer on Long Island: A case-control study. *Am J Epidemiol.* 2003; 158(1): 47–58.

50. O'Brien KM, Sandler DP, Taylor JA, Weinberg CR. Serum vitamin D and risk of breast cancer within five years. *Environ Health Perspect.* 2017; 125(7):077004. https://doi.org/10.1289/EHP943.

51. US Nuclear Regulatory Commission. https://www.nrc.gov/about-nrc /radiation/around-us/doses-daily-lives.html (Date accessed August 1, 2019).

52. National Institute of Environmental Health Sciences. Breast Cancer Risk and Environmental Factors. https://www.niehs.nih.gov/health/materials /environmental (Date accessed August 1, 2019).

53. Yaffe MJ and Mainprize JG. Risk of radiation-induced breast cancer from mammographic screening. *Radiology.* 2011; 258(1): 98–105.

54. Wells CL, Slanetz PJ, Rosen MP. Mismatch in breast and detector size during screening and diagnostic mammography results in increased patient radiation dose. *Acad Radiol.* 2014; 21(1): 99–103.

Chapter 3

1. Cardona RA and Ritchie EC. U.S. Military enlisted accession mental health screening: History and current practice. *Mil Med.* 2007; 172: 31–35.

2. Reiser SJ. The emergence of the concept of screening for disease. *Milbank Mem Fund Q Health Soc.*1978; 56(4): 403–425.

3. Hollier LM, Sheffield JS, Wendel GD. State laws regarding prenatal syphilis screening in the United States. *Am J Obstet Gynecol.* 2003; 189(4): 1178–1183.

4. *Reducing the Odds: Preventing Perinatal Transmission of HIV in the United States.* Washington, DC: National Academies Press, 1999. https://www.ncbi.nlm .nih.gov/books/NBK230552/ (Date accessed May 28, 2019).

5. Breslow L. An historical review of multiphasic screening. *Prev Med.* 1973; 2: 177–196.

6. Brief History of Newborn Screening. https://www.nichd.nih.gov/health/topics/newborn/conditioninfo/histor (Date accessed May 28, 2019).

7. Thorner RM and Remein QR. *Principles and Procedures in the Evaluation of Screening for Disease.* Washington, DC: Government Printing Office; 1961 (Public Health monograph no. 67). (Public Health Service publication no. 846).

8. Wilson JMG and Jungner G. *Principles and Practice of Screening for Disease.* Public Health Papers No. 34. Geneva, Switzerland: World Health Organization, 1968.

9. Harris R, Sawaya GF, Moyer VA, Calonge N. Reconsidering the criteria for evaluating proposed screening programs: Reflections from 4 current and former members of the U.S. Preventive Services Task Force. *Epidemiol Rev.* 2011; 33: 20–35.

10. U.S. Preventive Services Taskforce. https://www.uspreventiveservicestaskforce.org/Page/Name/recommendations (Date accessed May 23, 2019).

11. World Health Organization. Screening. https://www.who.int/cancer/prevention/diagnosis-screening/screening/en/ (Date accessed May 23, 2019).

12. Press N. Genetic testing and screening. In Crowley M (ed.). *From Birth to Death and Bench to Clinic: The Hastings Center Bioethics Briefing Book for Journalists, Policymakers, and Campaigns.* Garrison, NY: The Hastings Center, 2008, pp. 73–78.

Chapter 4

1. Worldwide Cancer Data. Global Cancer Statistics for the Most Common Cancers. World Cancer Research Fund. https://www.wcrf.org/dietandcancer/cancer-trends/worldwide-cancer-data (Date accessed June 29, 2019).

2. World Health Organization. Cancer. https://www.who.int/news-room/fact-sheets/detail/cancer (Date accessed June 29, 2019).

3. GBD 2015 Risk Factors Collaborators. Global, regional, and national comparative risk assessment of 79 behavioural, environmental and occupational, and metabolic risks or clusters of risks, 1990–2015: A systematic analysis for the Global Burden of Disease Study 2015. *Lancet.* 2016; 388(10053): 1659–1724.

4. World Health Organization. Cervical Cancer. https://www.who.int/cancer/prevention/diagnosis-screening/cervical-cancer/en/ (Date accessed May 24, 2019).

5. American Cancer Society Screening Guidelines for the Early Detection of Cancer. https://www.cancer.org/healthy/find-cancer-early/cancer-screening-guidelines/american-cancer-society-guidelines-for-the-early-detection-of-cancer.html (Date accessed May 24, 2019).

6. World Health Organization. Guidelines for Screening and Treatment of Precancerous Lesions for Cervical Cancer Prevention. 2013. https://apps.who.int/iris/bitstream/handle/10665/94830/9789241548694_eng.pdf;jsessionid=C6A2F0F130BA9ECDD110C67546B18986?sequence=1 (Date accessed June 17, 2019).

7. Ibid.

8. National Cancer Institute. HPV and Pap Testing. https://www.cancer.gov /types/cervical/pap-hpv-testing-fact-sheet (Date accessed May 24, 2019).

9. Gradissimo A and Burk RD. Molecular tests potentially improving HPV screening and genotyping for cervical cancer prevention. *Expert Rev Mol Diagn.* 2017; 17(4): 379–391.

10. Sankaranarayanan R, Nene BM, Shastri SS, et al. HPV Screening for cervical cancer in rural India. *N Engl J Med.* 2009; 360: 1385–1394.

11. Sherman ME, Lorinca AT, Scott DR, et al. Baseline cytology, human papilloma virus testing, and risk for cervical neoplasia: A 10-year cohort analysis. *J Natl Cancer Inst.* 2003; 95: 46–52.

12. Drolet M, Benard E, Perez N, Brisson M, on behalf of the HPV Vaccination Impact Study Group. Population-level impact and herd effects following the introduction of human papillomavirus vaccination programmes: Updated systematic review and meta-analysis. *Lancet.* June 26, 2019. http://doi.org/10.1016 /S0140-6736(19)30298-3.

13. World Health Organization. Cervical Cancer. https://www.who.int /reproductivehealth/topics/cancers/en/ (Date accessed May 23, 2019).

14. Stenson KM. Epidemiology and Risk Factors for Head and Neck Cancer. https://www.uptodate.com/contents/epidemiology-and-risk-factors-for -head-and-neck-cancer (Date accessed June 13, 2019).

15. World Health Organization. Global Data on the Incidence of Oral Cancer. https://www.who.int/oral_health/publications/cancer_maps/en/ (Date accessed June 13, 2019).

16. Macrae FA. Colorectal Cancer: Epidemiology, Risk Factors, and Protective Factors. https://www.uptodate.com/contents/colorectal-cancer-epidemiology-risk -factors-and-protective-factors (Date accessed June 13, 2019).

17. Colorectal Cancer: Epidemiology, Risk Factors, and Protective Factors. https://seer.cancer.gov/data/seerstat/nov2015/ (Date accessed June 17, 2019).

18. Siegel RL, Miller KD, Jemal A. Cancer statistics, 2019. *Cancer J Clin.* 2019; 69(1): 7.

19. Liang Z and Richards R. Virtual colonoscopy vs optical colonoscopy. *Expert Opin Med Diagn.* 2010; 4(2): 159–169. https://doi.org/10.1517/1753005100 3658736.

20. American Cancer Society Screening Guidelines for the Early Detection of Cancer, https://www.cancer.org/healthy/find-cancer-early/cancer-screening-guidelines /american-cancer-society-guidelines-for-the-early-detection-of-cancer.html

21. Colorectal Cancer Screening Tests. http://www.cdc.gov/cancer/colorectal /basic_info/screening/tests.htm (Date accessed June 17, 2019).

22. Ransohoff DF. How much does colonoscopy reduce colon cancer mortality? *Ann Inter Med.* 2009; 150(1): 50–52.

23. Siegel R, Miller KD, Jemal A. Cancer statistics, 2015. *CA Cancer J Clin.* 2015; 65: 5–29.

24. Global Burden of Disease Cancer Collaboration. Global, regional, and national cancer incidence, mortality, years of life lost, years lived with disability,

and disability-adjusted life-years for 32 cancer groups, 1990 to 2015: A systematic analysis for the global burden of disease study. *JAMA Oncol.* 2016; 3: 524–548.

25. Albertsen PC, Hanley JA, Fine J. 20-year outcomes following conservative management of clinically localized prostate cancer. *JAMA.* 2005; 293: 2095–2101.

26. Ferlay J, Soerjomataram I, Dikshit R, et al. Cancer incidence and mortality worldwide: Sources, methods and major patterns in GLOBOCAN 2012. *Int J Cancer.* 2015; 136: E359–E386.

27. Pernar CH, Ebot EM, Wilson KM, Mucci LA. The epidemiology of prostate cancer. *Cold Spring Harb Perspect Med.* 2018; 8: a030361. https://doi.org/10.1101/cshperspect.a030361.

28. Zhou XF, Ding ZS, Liu NB. Allium vegetables and risk of prostate cancer: Evidence from 132,192 subjects. *Asian Pac J Cancer Prev.* 2013; 14: 4131–4139.

29. Martin RM, Donovan JL, Turner EL, et al. Effect of a low-intensity PSA-based screening intervention on prostate cancer mortality. *JAMA.* 2018; 319(9): 883. https://doi.org/10.1001/jama.2018.0154.

30. Ong MS and Mandl KD. Trends in prostate-specific antigen screening and prostate cancer interventions 3 years after the U.S. Preventive Services Task Force recommendation. *Ann Intern Med.* 2017; 166(6): 451–452.

31. Moyer VA. U.S. Preventive Services Task Force. Screening for prostate cancer: U.S. Preventive Services Task Force recommendation statement. *Ann Intern Med.* 2012; 157:120–134.

32. American Cancer Society Screening Guidelines for the Early Detection of Cancer, https://www.cancer.org/healthy/find-cancer-early/cancer-screening-guidelines/american-cancer-society-guidelines-for-the-early-detection-of-cancer.html

33. Lung Cancer Screening. https://www.uspreventiveservicestaskforce.org/Page/Document/UpdateSummaryFinal/lung-cancer-screening (Date accessed June 29, 2019).

34. Lung Screening Trial Research Team, Aberle DR, Adams AM, Berg CD, et al. Reduced lung-cancer mortality with low-dose computed tomographic screening. *N Engl J Med.* 2011; 365(5): 395–409.

35. American Cancer Society Screening Guidelines for the Early Detection of Cancer,https://www.cancer.org/healthy/find-cancer-early/cancer-screening-guidelines/american-cancer-society-guidelines-for-the-early-detection-of-cancer.html

36. Wegwarth O, Schwartz LM, Woloshin S, et al. Do physicians understand cancer screening statistics? A national survey of primary care physicians in the United States. *Ann Intern Med.* 2012; 156 (5): 340–349.

Chapter 5

1. Picard JD. History of mammography. *Bull Acad Natl Med.* 1998; 182(8): 1613–1620.

2. Bassett LW and Gold RH. The evolution of mammography. *AJR Am J Roentgenol.* 1988; 150: 493–498.

3. Gold RH, Bassett LW, Widoff BE. Highlights from the history of mammography. *Radiographics.* 1990; 10: 1111–1131.

4. Elmore JG, Barton MB, Moceri VM, et al. Ten-year risk of false positive screening mammograms and clinical breast exam examinations. *N Engl J Med.* 1998; 338: 1089–1096.

5. Smith-Bindman R, Chu PW, Miglioretti DL, et al. Comparison of screening mammography in the United States and the United Kingdom. *JAMA.* 2003; 290: 2129–2137.

6. Kerlikowske KK and Barclay J. Outcomes of modern screening mammography. *J Natl Can Inst Mono.* 1997; 22: 105–111.

7. Houssami N. Overdiagnosis of breast cancer in population screening: Does it make breast screening worthless? *Cancer Biol Med.* 2017; 14(1): 1–8.

8. Biesheuvel C, Barratt A, Howard K, et al. Effects of study methods and biases on estimates of invasive breast cancer overdetection with mammography screening: A systematic review. *Lancet Oncol.* 2007; 8: 1129–1138.

9. Lauby-Secretan B, Scoccianti C, Loomis D, et al. Breast-cancer screening–viewpoint of the IARC Working Group. *N Engl J Med.* 2015; 372: 2353–2358.

10. Jørgensen KJ, Gøtzsche PC, Kalager M, et al. Breast cancer screening in Denmark: A cohort study of tumor size and overdiagnosis. *Ann Intern Med.* 2017; 166(5): 313–323.

11. Gøtzsche PC and Jørgensen KJ. Screening for breast cancer with mammography. *Cochrane Database Syst Rev.* 2013; Issue 6. Art. No.: CD001877. https://doi.org/10.1002/14651858.CD001877.pub5.

12. The Mammography Quality Standards Act Final Regulations: Preparing for MQSA Inspections: Final Guidance for Industry and FDA. https://www.fda.gov/media/74027/download (Date accessed August 29, 2019).

13. Pisano ED, Gatsonis C, Hendrick E, et al. Diagnostic performance of digital versus film mammography for breast-cancer screening. *N Engl J Med.* 2005; 353: 1773–1783.

14. Roubidoux MA, Bailey JE, Wray LA, Helvie MA. Invasive cancers detected after breast cancer screening yielded a negative result: Relationship of mammographic density to tumor prognostic factors. *Radiology.* 2004; 230: 42–48.

15. Helvie MA. Digital mammography imaging: Breast tomosynthesis and advanced applications. *Radiol Clin North Am.* 2010; 48(5): 917–929.

16. Good WF, Abrams GS, Catullo VJ, et al. Digital breast tomosynthesis: A pilot observer study. *Am J Roentgenol.* 2008; 190: 865–869.

17. Gur D, Abrams GS, Chough DM, et al. Digital breast tomosynthesis: Observer performance study. *Am J Roentgenol.* 2009; 193: 586–591.

18. Conant ER, Harlow WE, Herschorn SD, et al. Association of digital breast tomosynthesis vs digital mammography with cancer detection and recall rates by age and breast density. *JAMA Oncol.* 2019; 5(5): 635–642.

19. Bakker MF, de Lange SV, Pijnappel RM, et al. Supplemental MRI screening for women with extremely dense breast tissue. *N Engl J Med*. 2019; 381: 2091–2102.

20. Saslow D, Boetes C, Burke W, et al. American Cancer Society guidelines for breast screening with MRI as an adjunct to mammography. *CA Cancer J Clin*. 2007; 57: 75–89.

21. Brem RF, Tabar LK. Rapelyea JA, et al. Assessing improvement in detection of breast cancer with three-dimensional automated breast US in women with dense breast tissue: The SomoInsight Study. *Radiology*. 2015; 274: 663–673.

22. Thigpen D, Kappler A, Brem R. The role of ultrasound in screening dense breasts—A review of the literature and practical solutions for implementation. *Diagnostics (Basel)*. 2018; 8(1): 20.

23. Breast Thermography. http://www.breastthermography.com/breast _thermography_mf.htm (Date accessed August 26, 2019).

24. Arora N, Martins D, Ruggerio D, et al. Effectiveness of a noninvasive digital infrared thermal imaging system in the detection of breast cancer. *Am J Surg*. 2008; 196(4): 523–526.

25. Broach RB, Geha R Englander BS, et al. A cost-effective handheld breast scanner for use in low-resource environments: A validation study. *World J Surg Oncol*. 2016; 14: 277. https://doi.org/10.1186/s12957-016-1022-2.

26. McDonald S, Saslow D, Alciati MH. Performance and reporting of clinical breast examination: A review of the literature. *CA Cancer J Clin*. 2004; 54: 345–361.

27. Ibid.

28. McKinney SM, Sieniek M, Godbole V, et al. International evaluation of an AI system for breast cancer screening. *Nature*. 2020; 577: 89–94.

Chapter 6

1. DeSantis CE, Ma J, Sauer AG, et al. Breast cancer statistics, 2017, racial disparity in mortality by state. *CA Cancer J Clin*. 2017; 67: 439–448.

2. Walter LC and Covinsky KE. Cancer screening in elderly patients. *JAMA*. 2001; 285: 2750–2756.

3. Reuben DB. Medical care for the final years of life: "When you're 83, it's not going to be 20 year." *JAMA*. 2009; 302: 2686–2694.

4. Irwig L, Barratt A, Salkeld G. *Review of the Evidence about the Value of Mammographic Screening in 40–49 year old women*. Sydney, Australia: NHMRC National Breast Cancer Centre, 1997.

5. Burnside ES, Trentham-Dietz A, Shafer CM, et al. Age-based versus risk-based mammography screening in women 40–49 years old: A cross-sectional study. *Radiology*. 2019; 292: 321–328.

6. Price ER, Keedy AW, Gidwaney R, et al. The potential impact of risk-based screening mammography in women 40–49 years old. *Am J Roentgenol*. 2015; 205: 1360–1364.

7. Neal CH, Rahman WT, Joe AI, et al. Harms of restrictive risk-based mammographic breast cancer screening. *Am J Roentgenol.* 2018; 210: 228–234.

8. Consensus Development Statement: *Breast Cancer Screening for Women Ages 40–49.* Bethesda, MD: National Institutes of Health. January 1997. https://consensus.nih.gov/1997/1997BreastCancerScreening103html.htm (Date accessed November 9, 2019).

9. Royce TJ, Hendrix LH, Stokes WA, et al. Cancer screening rates in individuals with different life expectancies. *JAMA Intern Med.* 2014; 174(10): 1558–1565.

10. Demb J, Abraham L, Miglioretti DL, et al. Screening mammography outcomes: Risk of breast cancer and mortality by comorbidity score and age. *J Natl Cancer Inst.* https://doi.org/10.1093/jnci/djz172.

11. Barratt A, Irwig L, Glasziou P, et al. Benefits, harms and costs of screening mammography in women 70 years and over: A systematic review. *Med J Australia.* 2002; 176: 266–271.

12. Braithwaite D, Walter LC, Izano M, Kerlikowske K. Benefits and harms of screening mammography by comorbidity and age: A qualitative synthesis of observational studies and decision analyses. *J Gen Intern Med.* 2015; 31(5): 561–572.

13. *SEER Cancer Statistics Factsheets: Breast Cancer.* Bethesda, MD, 2015. http://seer.cancer.gov/statfacts/html/breast.html (Date accessed October 21, 2019).

14. Coldman A and Phillips N. Incidence of breast cancer and estimates of overdiagnosis after the initiation of a population-based mammography screening program. *CMAJ.* 2013; 185(10): E492–E498. https://doi.org/10.1503/cmaj.121791.

15. Garcia-Aleniz X, Hernan MA, Logan RW, et al. Continuation of annual screening mammography and breast cancer mortality in women over than 70 years. *Ann Intern Med.* 2020; https://doi.org/10.7326/M18-1199.

16. Parise C and Caggiano V. Breast cancer mortality among Asian-American women in California: Variation according to ethnicity and tumor subtype. *J Breast Cancer.* 2016; 19(2): 112–121.

17. Richardson LC, Henley J, Miller J, et al. Patterns and trends in black-white differences in breast cancer incidence and mortality—United States, 1999–2013. *MMWR.* 2016; 65(40): 1093–1098.

18. Ibid.

19. Centers for Disease Control and Prevention. Breast Cancer Rates among Black Women and White Women. 2016. https://www.cdc.gov/cancer/dcpc/research/articles/breast_cancer_rates_women.htm (Date accessed October 23, 2019).

20. Power EJ, Chin ML, Haq MM. Breast cancer incidence and risk reduction in the Hispanic population. *Cureus.* 2018; 10(2): e2235. https://doi.org/10.7759/cureus.2235.

21. Blanchard K, Colbert JA, Puri D, et al. Mammographic screening: Patterns of use and estimated impact on breast carcinoma survival. *Ann Intern Med.* 2004; 101(3): 495–507.

22. Centers for Disease Control. Use of mammography among women aged 40 and over, by selected characteristics: United States, selected years 1987–2015. https://www.cdc.gov/nchs/hus/contents2018.htm#Table_033 (Date accessed November 8, 2019).

23. Curtis E, Quale C, Haggstrom D, Smith-Bindman R. Racial and ethnic differences in breast cancer survival: How much is explained by screening, tumor severity, biology, treatment, comorbidities, and demographics? *Cancer.* 2008; 112(1): 171–180.

24. Noone AM, Howlader N, Krapcho M, et al., editors. SEER Cancer Statistics Review, 1975–2016. Table 4.18. Cancer of the female breast (invasive): Age-adjusted rates and trends by race/ethnicity. Bethesda, MD: National Cancer Institute, 2019. http://seer.cancer.gov/csr/1975_2016/ (Date accessed November 8, 2019).

25. American Cancer Society. *Breast Cancer Facts and Figures 2019–2020.* Atlanta, GA: American Cancer Society, 2019.

26. Ramjan L, Cotton A, Algoso M, Peters K. Barriers to breast and cervical cancer screening for women with physical disability: A review. *Women Health.* 2016; 56(2): 141–156.

27. Center for Disease Control and Prevention. It's Your Life. No one can protect it better than you. Know the facts about breast cancer screening. https://www.cdc.gov/ncbddd/disabilityandhealth/righttoknow/documents/tipsheetseng.pdf (Date accessed November 8, 2019).

28. Gigerenzer G. *Reckoning with Risk.* London: Penguin, 2002.

29. Thornton H, Edwards A, Baum M. Women need better information about routine mammography. *BMJ.* 2003; 327(7406): 101–103.

30. Alexandraki I and Mooradian A. Barriers related to mammography use for breast cancer screening among minority women. *J Natl Med Assoc.* 2010; 102: 206–218.

31. Miller BC, Bowers JM, Payne JB, Moyer A. Barriers to mammography screening among racial and ethnic minority women. *Soc Sci Med.* 2019; 239: 1–18. https://doi.org/10.1016/j.socscimed.2019.112494.

32. Croft E, Barratt A, Butow P. Information about tests for breast cancer: What are we telling people. *J Fam Practice.* 2002; 51: 858–860.

33. Jorgensen KJ and Gotzsche PC. Presentation of websites of possible benefits and harms from screening for breast cancer: Cross sectional study. *Brit Med J.* 2004; 328: 148–151.

34. Colby SL and Ortman JM. *Projections of the size and composition of the US Population: 2014 to 2060.* Report P25-1143. Washington, DC: US Census Bureau, 2015.

35. Qaseem A, Lin JS, Reem A, et al. Screening for breast cancer in average-risk women: A guidance statement from the American College of Physicians. *Ann Intern Med.* 2019; 170: 547–560.

36. Lee CH, Dershaw DD, Kopans D, et al. Breast cancer screening with imaging: Recommendations from the Society of Breast Imaging and the ACR on the

use of mammography, breast MRI, breast ultrasound, and other technologies for the detection of clinically occult breast cancer. *J Am Coll Radiol.* 2010; 7(1): 18–27.

Chapter 7

1. Shapiro S, VenetWL, Strax P, et al. *Periodic screening for breast cancer: The Health Insurance Plan Project and its sequelae, 1963–1983.* Baltimore: Johns Hopkins University Press, 1988.

2. Shapiro S, Venet W, Strax P, et al. Periodic screening for breast cancer: The HIP randomized controlled trial Health Insurance Plan. *J Natl Cancer Inst Monograph.* 1997; 22: 27–30.

3. Shaprio S, Strax P, Venet L, et al. Periodic breast cancer screening in reducing mortality from breast cancer. *JAMA.* 1971; 1777–1785.

4. Culliton BJ. Breast cancer: Second thoughts about routine mammography. *Science.* 1976; 193: 555–558.

5. Seidman H, Gleb SK, Silverberg E, et al. Survival experience in the Breast Cancer Detection Demonstration Project. *CA Cancer J Clin.* 1987; 37: 258–290.

6. Smart CA, Byrne CA, Smith RA. Twenty-year follow up of the breast cancers diagnosed during the Breast Cancer Detection Demonstration Project. *CA Cancer J Clin.* 1997; 47: 134–149.

7. Bailar JC, III. Mammography: A contrary view. *Ann Int Med.* 1976; 84: 77–84.

8. Greenberg DA. X-ray mammography—Background to a decision. *N Engl J Med.* 1976; 295: 739–740.

9. Andersson I, Aspegren K, Janzon L, et al. Mammographic screening and mortality from breast cancer: The Malmo Mammographic Screening Trial. *Br Med J.* 1988; 297: 943–948.

10. Frisell J, Lidbrink E, Hellstrom L, et al. Follow up after 11 years: Update of mortality results I the Stockholm Mammographic Screening Trial. *Breast Cancer Res Treat.* 1997; 45: 263–270.

11. Bjurstam N, Bjorneld L, Duffy SW, et al. The Gothenburg Breast Screening Trial: First results on mortality, incidence, and mode of detection for women ages 39–49 years at randomization. *Cancer.* 1997; 80: 2091–2099.

12. Nystrom L, Rutqvist LE, Wall S, et al. Breast cancer screening with mammography: Overview of Swedish randomized trials. *Lancet.* 1993; 341: 973–978.

13. Roberts MM, Alexander FE, Anderson TJ, et al. Edinburgh trail of screening for breast cancer: Mortality at seven years. *Lancet.* 1990; 335: 241–246.

14. Alexander FE, Anderson TJ, Brown HK, et al. The Edinburgh randomized trial of breast cancer screening. *Br J Cancer.* 1994; 70: 542–548.

15. Miller AB, Baines CJ, To T, et al. Canadian national Breast Screening Study: 1. Breast cancer detection and death rates among women aged 40–49 years. *CMAJ.* 1992; 147: 1459–1476.

16. Miller AB, Baines CJ, To T, et al. Canadian national Breast Screening Study: 2. Breast cancer detection and death rates among women aged 50–59 years. *CMAJ.* 1992; 147: 1477–1488.

17. Lerner BH. Fighting the war on breast cancer: Debates over early detection, 1945 to the present. *Ann Int Med.* 1998; 129: 74–78.

18. Leitch AM. Breast cancer screening: Success amid conflict. *Surg Oncol Clin N Am.* 1999; 8: 657–672.

19. Elmore JG, Barton MB, Moceri VM, et al. Ten-year risk of false positive screening mammograms and clinical breast examinations. *N Engl J Med.* 1998; 338: 1089–1096.

20. Gotzsche PC and Olsen O. Is screening for breast cancer with mammography justifiable? *Lancet.* 2000; 355: 129–134.

21. Horton R. Screening mammography—An overview revisited. *Lancet.* 2001; 358: 1284–1285.

22. Olsen O and Gotzsche PC. Cochrane review on screening for breast cancer with mammography. *Lancet.* 2001; 358: 1340–1342.

23. Tabar L, Yen MF, Vitak B, et al. Mammography service screening and mortality in breast cancer patients: 20-year follow up before and after introduction of screening. *Lancet.* 2003; 361: 1405–1410.

24. Bjurstam N, Bjorneld L, Duffy SW, et al. The Gothenburg Breast Screening Trial: First results on mortality, incidence, and mode of detection for women ages 39–49 years at randomization. *Cancer.* 1997; 80: 2091–2099.

25. Tabar L, Vitak B, Chen HHT, et al. Beyond randomized controlled trials: Organized mammographic screening substantially reduces breast carcinoma mortality. *Cancer.* 2001; 91: 1724–1731.

Chapter 8

1. National Cancer Institute. https://www.cancer.gov/about-cancer/diagnosis -staging/prognosis/tumor-grade-fact-sheet (Date accessed December 20, 2019).

2. American Cancer Society. Breast Cancer Facts and Figures, 2017–2018. https://www.cancer.org/content/dam/cancer-org/research/cancer-facts-and -statistics/breast-cancer-facts-and-figures/breast-cancer-facts-and-figures-2017 -2018.pdf (Date accessed December 20, 2019).

3. Freeman MD, Gopman JM, Salzberg CA. The evolution of mastectomy surgical technique: Type of operation performed. *Br J Cancer.* 1948; 2: 7–13.6.

4. Zurrida S, Bassi F, Arnone P, et al. The changing face of mastectomy (from mutilation to aid to breast reconstruction). *Int J Surg Oncol.* 2011; 2011: 980158.

5. Patey DH and Dyson WH. The prognosis of carcinoma of the breast in relation to the type of the mastectomy performed. *Br J Cancer.* 1948; 2: 7–13.

6. ibid.

7. Freeman MD, Gopman JM, Salzberg CA. The evolution of mastectomy surgical technique: From mutilation to medicine. *Gland Surg.* 2018; 7(3): 308–315.

8. Kennedy CS and Miller E. Simple mastectomy for mammary carcinoma. *Ann Surg.* 1963; 57: 161–162.

9. Kaae S and Johansen H. Simple mastectomy plus postoperative irradiation by the method of McWhirter for mammary carcinoma. *Ann Surg.* 1969; 170(6): 895–899.

10. Hartmann LC, Schaid DJ, Woods JE, et al. Efficacy of bilateral prophylactic local recurrence, and nipple-areolar recurrence in the setting of nipple-sparing mastectomy: A meta-analysis and systematic review. *Ann Surg Oncol.* 2015; 22: 3241–3249.

11. De La Cruz L, Moody AM, Tappy EE, et al. Overall survival, disease-free survival, versus non-skin-sparing mastectomy for breast cancer: A meta-analysis of observational studies. *Ann Surg.* 2010; 251: 632–639.

12. Fisher B, Bauer M, Margolese R, et al. Five-year results of a randomized clinical trial comparing total mastectomy and segmental mastectomy with or without radiation in the treatment of breast cancer. *N Engl J Med.* 1985; 312: 665–673.

13. Veronesi U, Cascinelli N, Mariani L, et al. Twenty-year follow-up of a randomized study comparing breast-conserving surgery with radical mastectomy for early breast cancer. *N Engl J Med.* 2002; 347(16): 1227032.

14. Poggi MM, Danforth DN, Sciuto LC, et al. Eighteen-year results in the treatment of early breast carcinoma with mastectomy versus breast conservation therapy: The National Cancer Institute Randomized Trial. *Cancer.* 2003; 98(4): 697–702.

15. Lanitis S, Tekkis PP, Sgourakis G, et al. Comparison of skin-sparing mastectomy mastectomy in women with a family history of breast cancer. *Ann Surg.* 2010; 251: 632–639.

16. Yi M, Kronowitz SJ, Meric-Bernstam F, et al. Local, regional, and systemic recurrence rates in patients undergoing skin-sparing mastectomy compared with conventional mastectomy. *Cancer.* 2011; 117: 916–924.

17. Early Breast Cancer Trialists' Collaborative Group, Darby S, McGale P, et al. effect of radiotherapy after breast-conserving surgery on 10-year recurrence and 15-year breast cancer death: Meta-analysis of individual patient data for 10,801 women in 17 randomised trials. *Lancet.* 2011; 378: 1707–1716.

18. Van Maaren MC, de Munck L, de Bock GH, et al. 10 year survival after breast-conserving surgery plus radiotherapy compared with mastectomy in early breast cancer in the Netherlands: A population-based study. *Lancet Oncol.* June 22, 2016. https://doi.org/10.1016/S1470-2045(16)30067-5.

19. Smith BD, Jiang J, Shih YC, et al. Cost and complications of local therapies for early-stage breast cancer. *J Natl Cancer Inst.* 2017: 109(1). https://doi.org/10.1093/jnci/djw178.

20. Jvan Dongen JA, Voogd AC, Fentiman IS, et al. Long-term results of a randomized trial comparing breast-conserving therapy with mastectomy: European Organization for Research and Treatment of Cancer 10801 trial. *Natl Cancer Inst.* 2000; 92(14): 1143–1150.

21. Tuttle TM, Abbott A, Arrington A, Rueth N. The increasing use of prophylactic mastectomy in the prevention of breast cancer. *Curr Oncol Rep.* 2010; 12(1): 16–21.

22. Alaofi RK, Nassif MO, Al-Hajeili MR. Prophylactic mastectomy for the prevention of breast cancer: Review of the literature. *Avicenna J Med.* 2018; 8(3): 67–77.

23. Connell PP and Hellman S. Advances in radiotherapy and implications for the next century: A historical perspective. *Cancer Res.* 2009; 69(2). https://doi.org/10.1158/0008-5472.CAN-07-6871.

24. Streeter OE, Vicini FA, Keisch M, et al. MammoSite radiation therapy system. *Breast.* 2003; 12(6): 491–496.

25. Vargo JA, Verma V, Kim H, et al. Extended (5-year) outcomes of accelerated partial breast irradiation using MammoSite balloon brachytherapy: Patterns of failure, patient selection, and dosimetric correlates for late toxicity. *Int J Radiat Oncol Biol Phys.* 2014; 88(2): 285–291.

26. Rosenkranz KM, Tsui E, McCabe EB, et al. Increased rates of long-term complications after MammoSite brachytherapy compared with whole breast radiation therapy. *J Am Coll Surg.* 2013; 217(3): 497–502.

27. Lukong KE. Understanding breast cancer—The long and winding road. *BBA Clin.* 2017. 7: 64–77. https://doi.org/10.1016/j.bbacli.2017.01.001.

28. Lee LJ and Harris JR. Innovations in radiation therapy (RT) for breast cancer. *Breast.* 2009; (Suppl 3): S103–S111. https://doi.org/10.1016/S0960-9776(09)70284-X.

29. Gianfaldoni S, Gianfaldoni R, Wollina U, et al. An overview on radiotherapy: From its history to its current applications in dermatology. *Open Access Maced J Med Sci.* 2017; 5(4): 521–525. https://doi.org/10.3889/oamjms.2017.122.

30. Burnstein HJ. Adjuvant chemotherapy for HER2-negative breast cancer. Up-To-Date. November 2019. https://www.uptodate.com/contents/adjuvant-chemotherapy-for-her2-negative-breast-cancer (Date accessed December 30, 2019).

31. Sparano JA, Gray RJ, Makower DF, et al. Prospective validation of a 21-gene expression assay in breast cancer. *N Engl J Med.* 2015; 373: 2005–2014.

32. Peto R, Davies C, Godwin J, et al. Comparisons between different polychemotherapy regimens for early breast cancer: Meta-analyses of long-term outcome among 100,000 women in 123 randomised trials. *Lancet.* 2012; 379(9814): 432.

33. Quirke VM. Tamoxifen from failed contraceptive pill to best-selling breast cancer medicine: A case-study in pharmaceutical innovation. *Front Pharmacol.* 2017; 8: 620.

34. Early Breast Cancer Trialists' Collaborative Group, Davies C, Godwin J, et al. Relevance of breast cancer hormone receptors and other factors to the efficacy of adjuvant tamoxifen: Patient-level meta-analysis of randomized trials. *Lancet.* 2011; 378: 771–784.

35. Davies C, Pan H, Godwin J, et al. Long-term effects of continuing adjuvant tamoxifen to 10 years versus stopping at 5 years after diagnosis of oestrogen

receptor-positive breast cancer: ATLAS, a randomized trial. *Lancet.* 2013; 381: 805–816.

36. Fabian CJ, Kimler BF. Selective estrogen-receptor modulators for primary prevention of breast cancer. *J Clin Oncol.* 2005; 23(8): 1644–1655.

37. Conzen SD. Managing the side effects of tamoxifen. Up-To-Date. November 2019. https://www.uptodate.com/contents/managing-the-side-effects-of-tamoxifen (Date accessed December 20, 2019).

38. Day R, Ganz PA, Costantion JP. Tamoxifen and depression: More evidence from the National Surgical Adjuvant Breast and Bowel Project's Breast Cancer Prevention (P-1) Randomized Study. *J Natl Cancer Inst.* 2001; 93(21): 1615–1623.

39. Simpson D, Curran MP, Perry CM. D. Letrozole: A review of its use in postmenopausal women with breast cancer. *Drugs.* 2004; 64(11): 1213–1230.

40. Baum M. The ATAC (Arimidex, Tamoxifen, alone or in combination) adjuvant breast cancer trial in postmenopausal patients: Factors influencing the success of patient recruitment. *Eur J Cancer.* 2002; 38: 1984–1986.

41. Cronin KA, Harlan LC, Dodd KW, et al. Population-based estimate of the prevalence of HER2 positive breast cancer tumors for early stage patients in the US. *Cancer Invest.* 2010; 28: 963–968.

42. Cameron P, Piccart-Gebhart MJ, Gelber RD, et al. 11 years' follow-up of trastuzumab after adjuvant chemotherapy in HER2-positive early breast cancer: Final analysis of the HERceptin Adjuvant (HERA) trial. *Lancet.* 2017; 389: 1195–1205.

43. Murthy RK, Loi S, Okines A, et al. Tucatinib, trastuzumab, and capecitabine for HER2 positive metastatic breast cancer. *N Engl J Med.* December 11, 2019. https://doi.org/10.1056/NEJMoa1914609

Chapter 9

1. Tinoco G, Warsch S, Cluck S, et al. Treating breast cancer in the 21st century: Emerging biological therapies. *J Cancer.* 2013; 4(2): 117–132.

2. Campbell PJ, Getz G, Korbel JD, et al. Pan-cancer analysis of whole genomes. *Nature.* 2020; 578: 82–93.

3. Mansoori B, Mohammadi A, Davudian S, et al. The different mechanisms of cancer drug resistance: A brief review. *Adv Pharm Bull.* 2017; 7: 339–348.

4. National Research Council. What is the Difference between Precision Medicine and Personalized Medicine? What about Pharmacogenomics? https://ghr .nlm.nih.gov/primer/precisionmedicine/precisionvspersonalized (Date accessed February 27, 2020).

5. Precision Medicine Initiative. https://obamawhitehouse.archives.gov/the -press-office/2015/01/30/fact-sheet-president-obama-s-precision-medicine-initiative (Date accessed February 26, 2020).

6. Lathe WC, Williams JM, Mangan ME, Karolchik D. Genomic data resources: Challenges and promises. *Nat Educ.* 2008; 1(3): 2.

7. The Human Genome Project. https://www.genome.gov/human-genome -project (Date accessed February 26, 2020).

8. Jain K. Applications of biochips: From diagnostics to personalized medicine. *Curr Opin Drug Discov Devel.* 2004; 7(3): 285–289.

9. National Cancer Institute. Targeted Cancer Therapies. https://www.cancer .gov/about-cancer/treatment/types/targeted-therapies/targeted-therapies -fact-sheet (Date accessed January 27, 2020).

10. Schlisky RL. Tumor-Agnostic Treatment for Cancer: An Expert Perspective. Cancer.Net. December 20, 2018. https://www.cancer.net/blog /2018-12/tumor-agnostic-treatment-cancer-expert-perspective (Date accessed January 29, 2020).

11. Riley RS, June CH, Langer R, Mitchell MJ. Delivery technologies for cancer immunotherapy. *Nat Rev Drug Discov.* 2019; 18(3): 175–196.

12. Cancer Research Institute. What Is Immunotherapy. https://www .cancerresearch.org/immunotherapy/what-is-immunotherapy?gclid= EAIaIQobChMI3NL3heWr5wIVBFYMCh1YzQ4hEAAYAiAAEgLTKPD_BwE (Date accessed January 30, 2020).

13. Bateman AC. Molecules in cancer immunotherapy: Benefits and side effects. *J Clin Pathol.* 2019; 72: 20–24.

14. Monoclonal Antibody Drugs for Cancer: How They Work. https://www .mayoclinic.org/diseases-conditions/cancer/in-depth/monoclonal-antibody/art -20047808 (Date accessed February 18, 2020).

15. Overview of Targeted Therapies for Cancer. https://www.mycancergenome .org/content/page/overview-of-targeted-therapies-for-cancer/ (Date accessed January 29, 2020).

16. Shiel WC. Medical Definition of T-Cell Depletion. https://www .medicinenet.com/script/main/art.asp?articlekey=11300 (Date accessed February 26, 2020).

17. National Cancer Institute, Targeted Cancer Therapies.

18. Madden, DL. From a patient advocate's perspective: Does cancer immunotherapy represent a paradigm shift? *Curr Oncol Rep.* 2018; 20: 8. https://doi .org/10.1007/s11912-018-0662-5.

19. Crowther MD, Dolton G, Legut M, et al. Genome-wide CRISPR–Case screening reveals ubiquitous T cell cancer targeting via the monomorphic MHC class I-related protein MR1. *Nat Immunol.* January 20, 2020. https://doi.org/10 .1038/s41590-019-0578-8.

20. Stemmer SM, Steiner M, Rizel, S, et al. Clinical outcomes in ER+ HER2 -node-positive breast cancer patients who were treated according to the Recurrence Score results: Evidence from a large prospectively designed registry. *NPJ Breast Cancer.* 2017; 3: 32. https://doi.org/10.1038/s41523-017-0033-7.

21. CRISPR Genome Editing Holds Back Triple-Negative Breast Cancer in Mice. https://www.genengnews.com/news/crispr-genome-editing-holds-back -triple-negative-breast-cancer-in-mice/ (Date accessed February 26, 2020).

Chapter 10

1. Subramani R and Lakshmanaswamy R. Complementary and alternative medicine and breast cancer. *Prog Mol Biol Transl Sci*. 2017; 151: 231–274.

2. National Center for Complementary and Integrative Health. https://www.nccih.nih.gov/about/nccih-facts-at-a-glance-and-mission (Date accessed June 10, 2020).

3. Office of Cancer Complementary and Alternative Medicine. https://cam.cancer.gov/cam_at_nci/default.htm (Date accessed June 10, 2020).

4. National Cancer Institute. Clinical Trials for Complementary or Alternative Medicine Procedure(s). https://www.cancer.gov/about-cancer/treatment/clinical-trials/cam-procedures (Date accessed June 10, 2020).

5. Greenlee H, DuPont-Reyes MJ, Balneaves LG, et al. Clinical practice guidelines on the evidence-based us of integrative therapies during and following breast cancer treatment. *CA Cancer J Clin*. 2017; 67: 194–232.

6. Eisenberg DM, Kessler RC, Foster C, et al. Unconventional medicine in the United States. Prevalence, costs, and patterns of use. *N Engl J Med*. 1993; 328(4): 246–252.

7. Gansler T, Kaw C, Crammer C, Smith T. A population-based study of prevalence of complementary methods use by cancer survivors: A report from the American Cancer Society's studies of cancer survivors. *Cancer*. 2008; 113: 1048.

8. Roberts CD, Baker F, Hann D, et al. Patient-physician communication regarding use of complementary therapies during cancer treatment. *J Psychosoc Oncol*. 2006; 23(4): 35–60.

9. Zaid H, Silbermann M, Amash A, et al. Medicinal plants and natural active compounds for cancer chemoprevention/chemotherapy. *Evid Based Complement Alternat Med*. 2017; 2017: 7952417. https://doi.org/10.1155/2017/7952417.

10. Buckner CA, Lafrenie RM, Denommee JA, et al. Complementary and alternative medicine use in patients before and after a cancer diagnosis. *Curr Oncol*. 2018; 25(4): e275–e281. https://doi.org/10.3747/co.25.3884.

Chapter 11

1. Holland JC. Psychological care of patients: Psycho-oncology's contribution. *J Clin Oncolo*. 2003; 23s: 253s–265s.

2. Chen M and Zhao L. Mapping breast cancer survivors' psychosocial coping along disease trajectory: A language approach. *J Health Psychol*. https://doi.org/10.1177/1359105320919893.

3. Sharma N, Purkayastha A. Factors affecting quality of life in breast cancer patients: A descriptive and cross-sectional study with review of literature. *J Midlife Health*. 2017; 8(2): 75–83.

4. Petticrew M, Bell R, Hunter D. Influence of psychological coping on survival and recurrence in people with cancer: Systematic review. *Br Med J.* 2003; 12: 319–330.

5. Lang-Rollin I and Berberich G. Psycho-oncology. *Dialogues Clin Neurosci.* 2018; 20(1): 13–22.

6. Jagsi R, Ward KC, Abrahamse PH, et al. Unmet need for clinician engagement regarding financial toxicity after diagnosis of breast cancer. *Cancer.* 2018; 124(18): 3668–3676.

Chapter 12

1. Hall JA, Roter DL, Rand CS. Communication of affect between patient and physician. *J Health Soc Behav.* 1981; 22: 18–30.

2. Katz, J. *The Silent World of Doctor and Patient.* New York: The Free Press, 1984.

3. Lerner, BH. *The Good Doctor.* Boston: Beacon Press, 2014.

4. Institute of Medicine, Committee on Improving the Quality of Cancer Care: Addressing the Challenges of an Aging Population. Patient-centered communication and shared decision making. In Levit L, Balogh E, Nass S, et al. (eds). *Delivering High-Quality Cancer Care: Charting a New Course for a System in Crisis.* Washington, DC: National Academies Press, 2013, chapter 3. https://www.ncbi .nlm.nih.gov/books/NBK202146/ (Date accessed March 27, 2020).

5. Berkman ND, Sheridan SL, Donahue KE, et al. Health literacy interventions and outcomes: An updated systematic review. *Evid Rep Technol Assess.* 2011; (199). https://www.ncbi.nlm.nih.gov/pmc/articles/PMC4781058/ (Date accessed March 27, 2020).

6. Ibid.

7. OHRI (Ottawa Hospital Research Institute). A to Z Inventory of Decision Aids. March 29, 2013. http://decisionaid.ohri.ca/AZinvent.php (Date accessed March 27, 2020).

8. Ofri D. *What Patients Say, What Doctors Hear.* Boston: Beacon Press, 2017.

9. Glyn E, Paul JB, Sheri P. Digital clinical encounters. *BMJ;* 2018; k2061. https://doi.org/10.1136/bmj.k2061.

10. Monden KR, Gentry L, Cox TR. Delivering bad news to patients. *Proc (Bayl Univ Med Cent).* 2016; 29(1): 101–102.

11. Ibid.

12. Stewart M, Brown JB, Donner A, et al. The impact of patient-centered care on outcomes. *J Fam Pract.* 2000; 49: 796–804.

13. Ha JF and Longnecker N. Doctor-patient communication: A review. *Oschner J.* 2010; 10: 38–43.

14. Greenlee H, Ernst E. What can we learn from Steve Jobs about complementary and alternative therapies? *Prev Med.* 2012; 54(1): 3–4.

15. Mauksch LB, Dugdale DC, Dodson S, Epstein R. Relationship, communication, and efficiency in the medical encounter: Creating a clinical model from a literature review. *Arch Intern Med.* 2008; 168: 1387–1395.

16. Tai-Seale M, McGuire TG, Zhang W. Time allocation in primary care office visits. *Health Serv Res.* 2007; 42(5): 1871–1894.

17. Naykky S, Ospina K, Phillips R, et al. Eliciting the patient's agenda-secondary analysis of recorded clinical encounters. *J Gen Intern Med.* 2018; https://doi.org/10.1007/s11606-018-4540-5.

18. Lerman C, Daly M, Walsh WP, et al. Communication between patients with breast cancer and health care providers. Determinants and implications. *Cancer.* 1992; 72: 2612–2620.

19. Ibid.

20. Personal communication from a breast cancer survivor.

21. Tongue JR, Epps HR, Forese LL. Communication skills for patient-centered care: Research-based, easily learned techniques for medical interviews that benefit orthopaedic surgeons and their patients. *J Bone Joint Surg Am.* 2005; 87: 652–658.

Chapter 13

1. Jongerius C, Russo S, Mazzocco K, Pravettoni G. Research-tested mobile apps for breast cancer care: Systematic review. *JMIR Mhealth Uhealth.* 2019; 7(2): e10930. https://doi.org/10.2196/10930.

2. National Cancer Institute. https://www.cancer.gov/about-cancer/treatment/clinical-trials/search/trial-guide#2 (Date accessed April 30, 2020).

Index

Note: Page numbers followed by *t* indicate tables and *f* indicate figures.

About the Author

Madelon L. Finkel, PhD, is a professor of population health sciences and director of the Office of Global Health Education at Weill Cornell Medicine of Cornell University. Her areas of interest include cancer epidemiology, environmental health, and women's health. Dr. Finkel is the author of over 100 peer-reviewed articles, book chapters, and 15 books on various public health topics, and she serves as contributing editor to several professional journals. Two of her books, *Understanding the Mammography Controversy: Science, Politics, and Breast Cancer Screening* (Praeger, 2005) and *Cancer Screening in the Developing World: Case Studies and Strategies from the Field* (2018), have won book awards.